The WONDERS of
NETTLES

Free Superfood and Health Care

Janice J. Schofield

SECOND EDITION

The intent of this book is solely informational and educational. It is not intended as medical advice. Though nettles, properly harvested, prepared, and cooked have been used by countless generations, allergies and contraindications exist and the author/publisher is not responsible for your use or misuse. Please consult your health care provider before using nettles, especially if pregnant, nursing, or with a known medical condition or prescribed medications.

PREFACE

In my New Zealand garden sits a simple sign: The Wonders of Nettles, appropriately planted in the stinging nettle patch. The nettles ring my garden, protecting it well from the voracious appetites of my four riding lawnmowers. The mowers are none other than my horses, who would lean on the garden netting and lop the heads off my cabbages and tomato plants- prior to the nettle fence. Today, nettle robustly deters my lawn-mowing steeds from garden-munching, plus yields a steady stream of free food and healthful fare for my family, neighbors, and guests.

Despite the endless gifts to humanity that nettles yield, they are often whacked, weeded, or poisoned. Nettle protects itself from browsers and can indeed sting the unwary. But don't be alarmed! Just be alert and aware. Learn to identify, harvest, and prepare nettles correctly (which is easy with this guide). You will find nettles a safe and sensational food and healing aid. Additionally, these superfoods are free from the wild or can be easily cultivated.

If carelessly handled, the worst that the vast majority of the world's nettles do is create a temporary stimulating irritation. But even the sting is not 'all bad.' Deliberately stinging oneself is a traditional healing aid for easing arthritic pain. So, relax. This book guides you step by step into the proper identification and use of a veritable power-food and family helper.

Keep in mind that temperate areas have a far longer nettle harvest season than northern latitudes. Consistently harvesting the greens stimulates regrowth and extends the harvest. Spring is, of course, the prime harvest season. As New Zealand descends into winter in late April to early May, I delight in migrating to

Alaska. And Homer, Alaska, is the town I consider to be one of the world's nettle capitals.

As hardy nettles emerge from the chilled earth, my friends and I celebrate the spring harvest ritual. We rediscover how our bodies crave this nutrient-dense green and eat nettles (together with wild Alaskan salmon) for breakfast, lunch, and dinner. New nettle creations evolve, and new recipes are shared.

Given the state of the world at present- with countless climate challenges, the Covid pandemic, economic fallouts, and rampant disease, I feel compelled to bring *The Wonders of Nettles* back into print (and e-book). The original version of *Nettles* (published by Keats Publishing/McGraw Hill in 1998) contained but one black and white illustration. This edition is vibrant with color photographs and expanded content.

Nettles are a gift to the world, and this labor of love is my gift to you. This project could continue endlessly as more and more nettle info is unearthed, but it is time now for nettles to help the world. My blog will have to serve to release additional recipes and tips. Follow along at:

https://www.athomewithjaniceschofieldeaton.com

ACKNOWLEDGEMENTS

Nettles exist on every continent (except Antarctica). And the love of nettles links a global family of enthusiasts. This book has truly been a planetary endeavor, with contributors sharing freely from Finland's nettled fields to Tasmania's highlands, the byways of Europe, the far reaches of Turkey and Brazil, and from Alaska to New Zealand. Countless individuals have assisted this book's unfolding, both in its original format released over two decades ago and this revised and expanded present edition.

Heartfelt thanks to all the friends, authors, and contributors to this testament to nettles. Since this project first began, I, like so many others, have experienced world-shaking changes. Remarriage. Relocation from Alaska to New Zealand. And loss: a fire that consumed countless documents and my herbal library. If any credits or references have been missed, please accept my apology. Please know you are loved and will be recognized in a future edition. Without the help of nettle enthusiasts worldwide, this ode to nettles would not be able to be shared.

Special recognition to my husband Barry Eaton for his love, patience, and encouragement during this nettle book's rebirth. Gratitude to 'computer guru' Sunil Bhatla for leaping my final hurdles of print to press. Thanks to my pre-reading and editing team, Louise Desclos, Kim Aspelund, Gayla Pedersen, Shelley Lipman, Robyn Martin, and Emily Willis. Blessings to Connie Taylor of Fathom Publishing for tips and encouragement.

Recognition to Sandra Preinl of Germany, Crystal Li of China, and Chani Petro of the USA for inspiration and contributions; to Nancy Lee-Evans, Charles Evans, Ellen Vande Visse, and Wendy Anderson for company and kitchen space during countless nettle creations; to Sue Ellen Christiansen, Darlene Hildebrand, and Marina Schaum for endless moral support; to Parvati, Jamie Gomer, Bryan Myers, Jane Bell, the late Steve Johnson, Shoshanna Sadow, Kevin Spelman, H. Reid Shaw, Susan Lie-Nielsen, Sarah Murnane, Julia Mulder, for all your help; to brew master Lasse Holmes of Homer Alaska, Sean Cullerton of Home Brew Shop, and Kathleen Brewer for assistance in creating the outrageous Stinger (and kudos to Colette Ireland for its name); to Andrew Pengelly, Henriette Kress and Robyn Klein for perceptive editing; to Dominique Collet for drawing from the heart; to Edye E. Groseclose for biochemical insights; to Marilyn J. Dick, Jan Hermse and Andreas Ryser for generously sharing nettle information; to Robin Hopper for nettlesome music, and Lia Fields for creating the tune to the ancient words; to Ken Osetrof for tracking down Australian details; to Mairiis Kilcher and the late Deiv Rector for originally opening my heart, and taste buds to nettles; to the Herbal Hall and nettle lovers worldwide for so willingly sharing your wisdom, recipes, stories and experiences; and most of all to nettle herself, for freely bestowing gifts on a planet that is not always grateful.

CONTENTS

THE WONDERS OF NETTLES

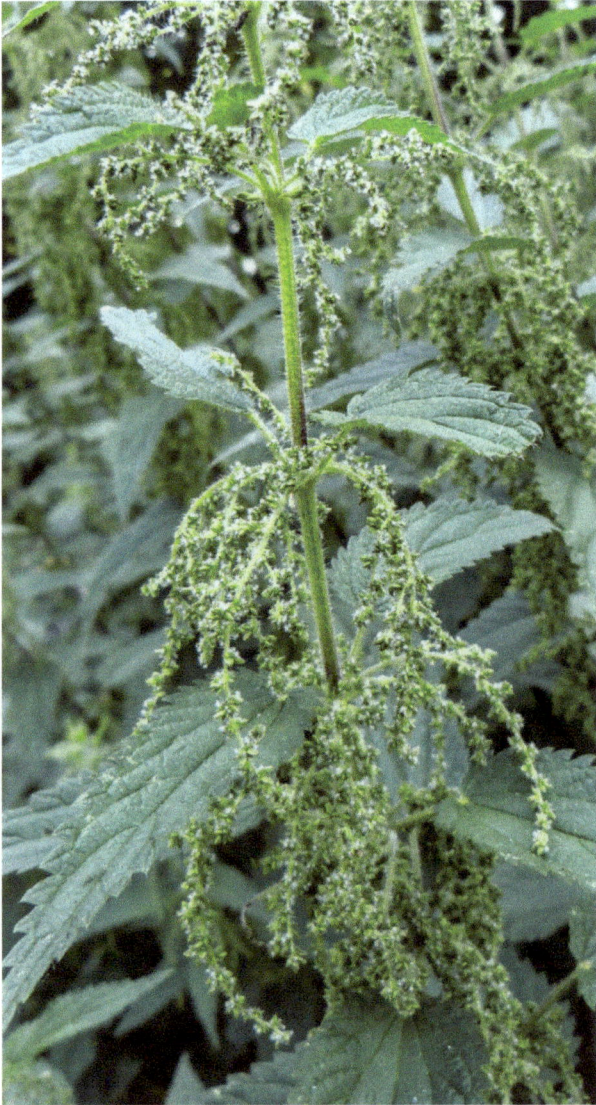

Chapter 1

Weed or Wonder?

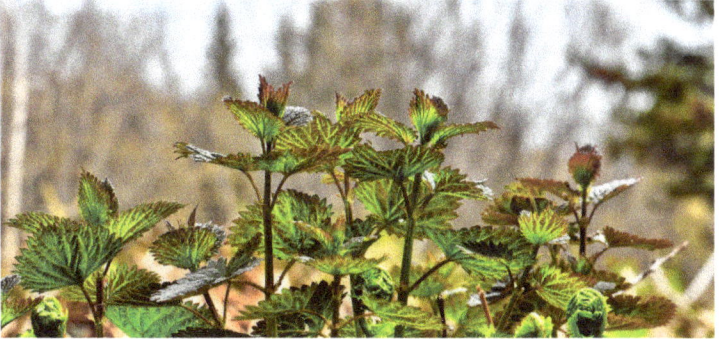

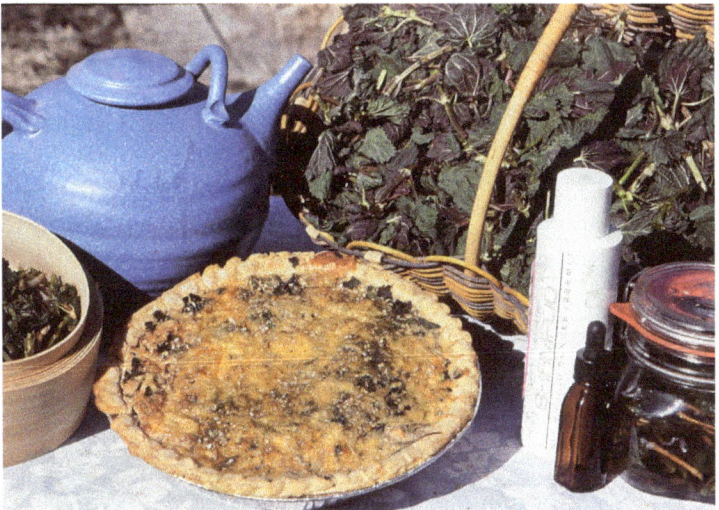

"What can be more hateful than the nettle?
Yet this plant simply abounds in remedies."
- Pliny

People who inadvertently tangle with stinging nettles quickly learn the error of their ways. Contacting the painful stinging hairs convinces many that they've encountered a despicable plant. This attitude is further reinforced by agricultural departments whose focus on cash crop cultivation leads them to scorn nettles as a 'noxious weed.'

Nettles do indeed have some weedlike characteristics. They feature both an unspectacular appearance (individual flowers are tiny) and the weedy habit of spreading globally, frequently turning up in well-populated or 'neglected' areas.

However, to refer to the common stinging nettles (*Urtica dioica*) and its many variations as 'noxious' (i.e., harmful to health) is most unfair. Though nettles temporarily sting the skin as a self-protective mechanism, they offer untold nourishment to body tissues. As indigenous people worldwide have long known, the shoots and leaves are an invaluable spring tonic and dietary delicacy. Roots also have multifaceted benefits (detailed in chapter four).

This book is a testament to the healing power and diverse uses of this simple cosmopolitan plant, a most amazing 'weed' and superfood. If unavailable for wild-harvesting, it well deserves to be deliberately cultivated.

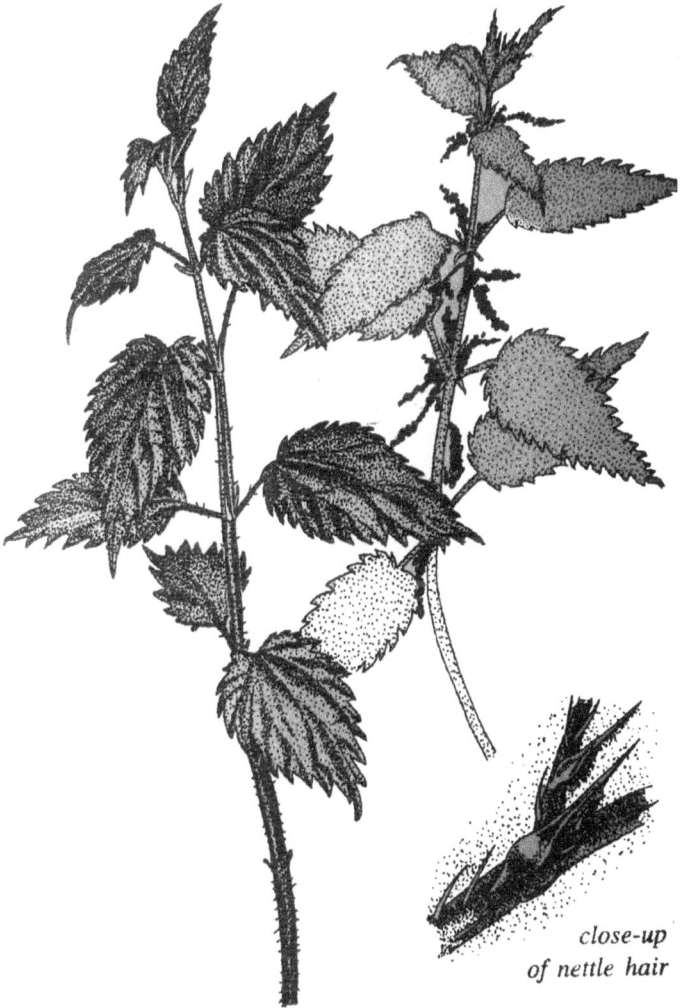

close-up
of nettle hair

Nettle *drawing by Dominique Collet*

Safety and Harvest

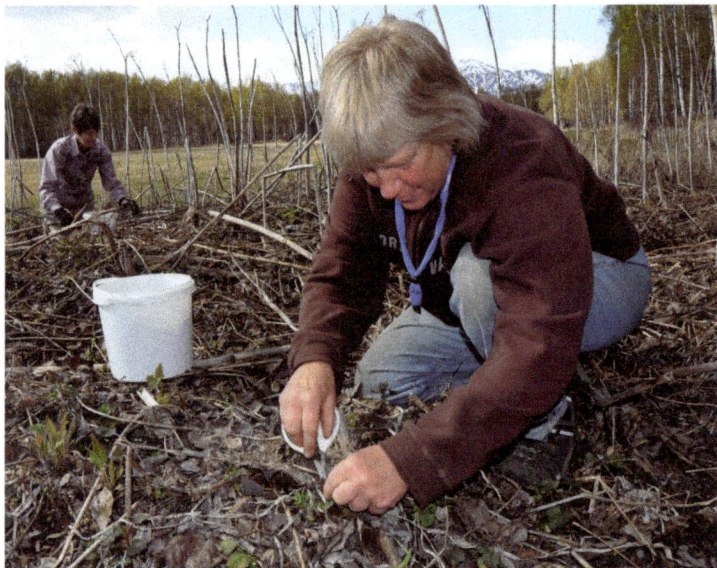

"This herb teaches us about paying attention."

– G.E. in Johnny's Selected Seeds catalog

Though safe when handled and identified correctly, nettles demand an attentive mind. This section addresses the identification of nettle, harvest guidelines, and how to evaluate quality if purchasing nettles from a shop.

Please read this chapter thoroughly before harvesting nettles. As shown in the photo, the forager in the rear uses gloves to avoid contact with the stinging hairs. Wendy Anderson, in the foreground, is deliberately picking nettles barehanded. The tall stalks surrounding this Alaskan nettle patch are cow parsnip

(*Heracleum lanatum*), a 'wild celery' whose juices can irritate the skin.

Note: Not everyone has suitable habitat available to wildcraft wild plants. Foragers intimately know the cleanliness of the habitat where their nettles are grown and the precise growth stage at harvest. Purchasers, on the other hand, need to develop skills to evaluate the quality of bought nettles.

Tips for Purchasing & Evaluating Dried Nettles

Health shops and natural food groceries typically stock nettle products as well as dried nettles in bulk. Develop your observational eye (and nose) and evaluate thoroughly before buying.

Properly dried nettles are a vibrant deep green with a pleasant earthy aroma. The presence of thick stems, large leaves, flowers, or seeds indicates nettles picked past their prime.

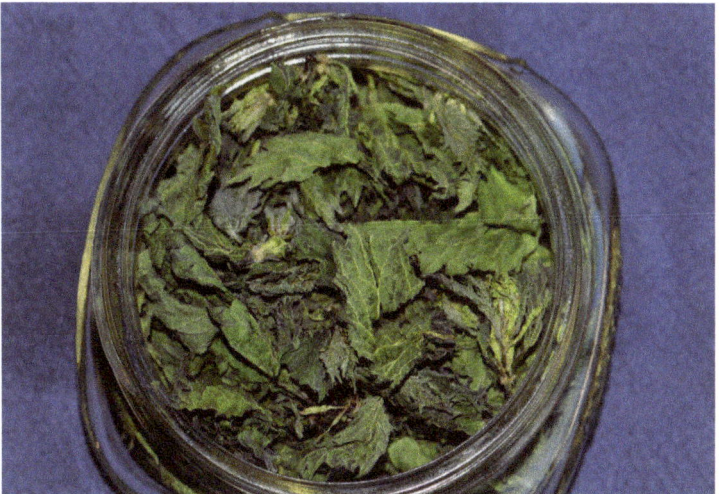

Fresh Nettles

An essential for many of the culinary recipes included in this book—fresh nettles can be challenging to purchase. (One exception is Turkey, where they are common in open-air markets.) Your most likely source for fresh nettles is to wild-harvest or cultivate them.

"Nettles are so well-known that they need no description: they may be found, by feeling, in the darkest night."

- Culpeper

Though touching stinging nettles is indeed one method of identifying the herb, conducting a visual botanical identification is far more pleasant and safe.

Nettles Worldwide

North American and European forages have a wide variety of species to safely use interchangeably—including *Urtica dioica*, *U. gracilis*, and *U. Lyallii*. Those living in New Zealand and Asia should consult the Dangers section later in this chapter.

Taming the Nettle

Even novices to plant identification will find the common stinging nettles easy to identify. If you miss keying to exact species, so long as you've positively identified the genus *Urtica*, you'll be in good company. We'll begin with a close look at *Urtica Lyallii* and then explore some of its variations.

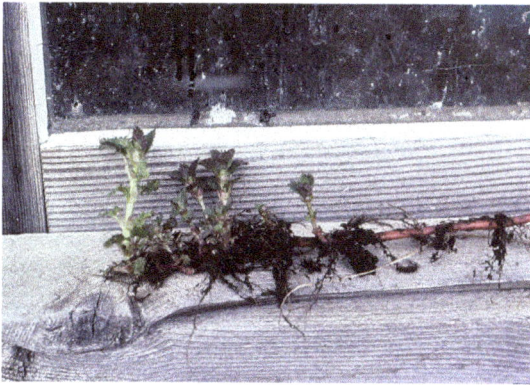

Urtica Lyallii is a perennial that regrows each year from its rootstock and its self-sown seed. Dig at the plant's base, and you will uncover a long rootstock that connects neighbor to neighbor.

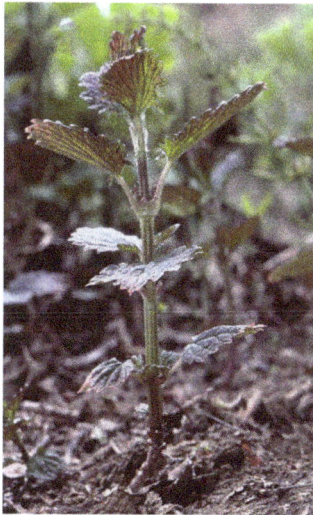

Urtica Lyallii, early spring phase

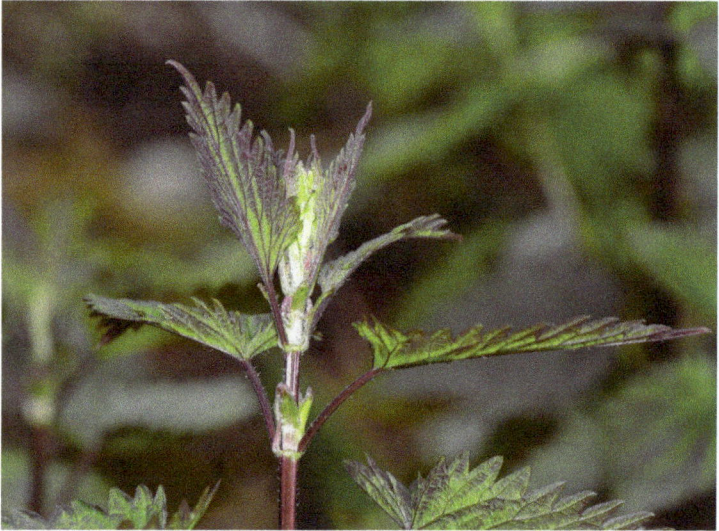

Note the fine, rigid hairs both on the square stems and on the leaves.

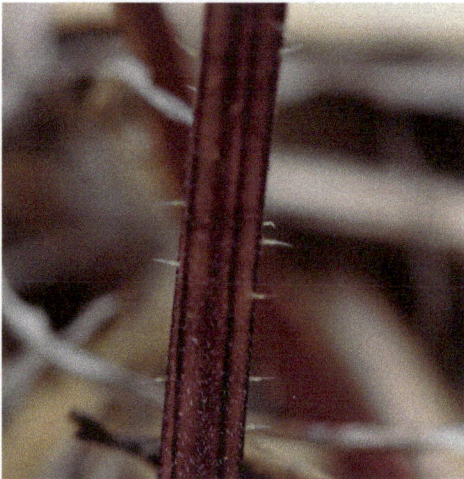

The hair base is swollen and contains the chemicals that cause stinging.

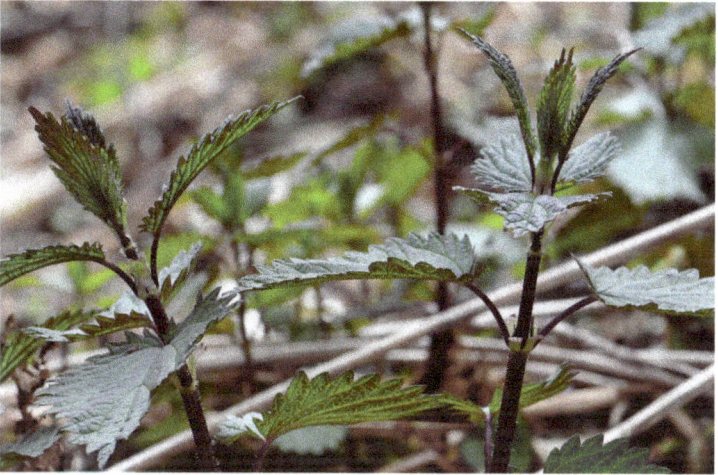

The leaves attach to the stems in an opposite (pair-like) arrangement and rotate as they ascend the stem. The leaves are coarsely toothed and ovate (approximately egg-shaped). The leaf base is commonly cordate (heart-shaped), although variations occur, including that of appearing truncated (sharply cut). The leaf tips end in a sharp point, either abruptly or with a bit of a taper.

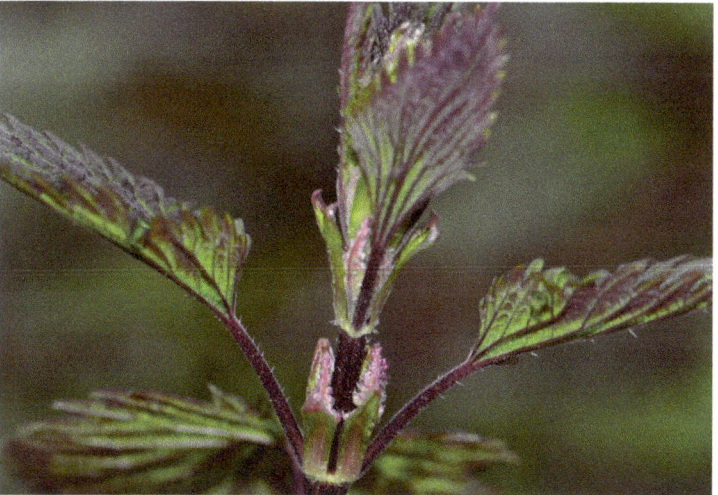

"The flowers of the stinging nettle," says Alaskan Mary Lee Plumb-Mentjes, "are most interesting for what they are not. They are not colorful or pretty. Like the flowers of many trees, they are green, dangling and wind-pollinated, having no relationship to the world of insects, birds or bats."

The minute greenish-to-purple catkins appear in early to mid-summer. (Catkins are hanging flower spikes that are usually wind-pollinated, unisex and lacking petals.) Nettle catkins grow from the axils (where leaves join the stem) and mature from the plant's base to the tip.

Many nettle species, including *Urtica Lyallii* (previous page, bottom), have monoecious flowers, i.e., both male and female flowers on the same plant. The flowers are the drooping clusters (shown here emerging at axils).

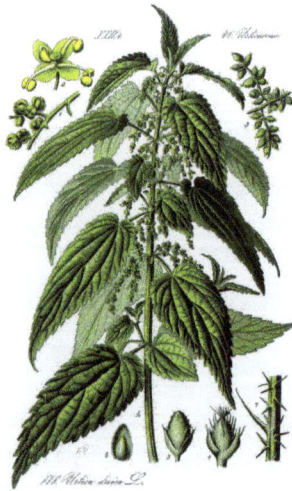

Urtica dioica has male and female flowers generally borne on separate plants. Males are erect and bear stamens (left); the longer drooping female flowers bear pistils (right).[1]

The species name stems from *dioecious*, which translates as 'two houses.' The male anthers use coiled springs to launch pollen into the air and, aided by the wind, fertilize the female stigma (right).

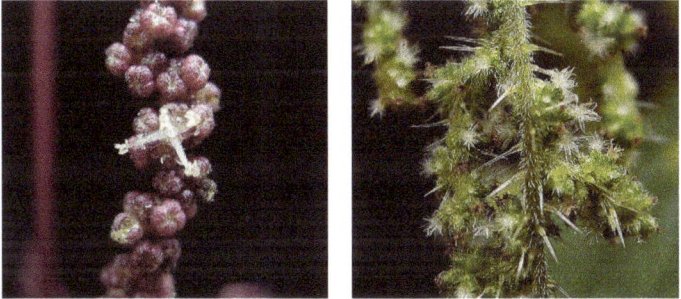

Photographs by Frank Vincentz[2]

Nettle Seeds

Nettle seeds are tiny and germinate minute seedlings that slowly become recognizable as nettle plants. Mature nettle plants can average 3 to 6 feet high (approximately 1 to 1.8 meters). Size variability exists with species, growing conditions, and region.

Novices find it easiest to identify plants positively when in flower or seed. And then can follow their targeted plant throughout the entire season, mastering recognition in all stages of growth. Due to nettle's propensity for stinging, it gives clues to its identity even when young.

Difference Between Common *Urtica* Species

Differences between the common North American and European nettle species are relatively minor. *Urtica Lyallii* (sometimes classified as *U. dioica*, subspecies *Lyallii*) bears broader, shorter leaves with deeper teeth than the longer, narrower-leaf *U. gracilis* (a.k.a. *U. dioica*, subspecies *gracilis*).

U. Lyallii ranges on the west coast of the United States from California to Alaska.

U. dioica, a widely naturalized American species, originates from Europe and Asia. Its leaves are mostly ovate leaves and taper to a sharp point. They may be heart-shaped and abruptly cut at the base. *U. dioica* also has a Scandinavian subspecies *U. sondenii* which is stingless.

U. urens (often called dwarf nettle) is an annual that ranges from 3 inches high to more than a foot in height (.30 meters).

There are approximately 50 *Urtica* species worldwide. If you need help identifying your area's nettle species, see a university botanist, a local plant expert, or a Flora of your bioregion. (A Flora contains the species found within a region, along with their identification details.)

Name Derivation

The genus name *Urtica* derives from the Latin *uro*, 'to burn.' It aptly describes the sensation that occurs when one physically contacts the fresh plant. The common word 'nettle' stems from the Dutch *netel*, meaning a needle, and refers to the hairs' hypodermic-like action. Nettles are also associated with 'nets,' as their fibers were reverse-wrapped to form a strong string and woven into fishing nets. During the world wars, many soldiers wore nettle uniforms.

Range and Habitat of *Urtica* Species

Nettles range throughout the temperate zone. *Urtica dioica* is indigenous to the British Isles, northern Europe, and Asia. *U. gracilis* is considered native to North America. Both species have established themselves in Australia and New Zealand.

Within a plant's range, knowing its preferred habitat helps you predict where it will occur. Nettles thrive in moist areas, old garden sites, and mixed woods. When my small barn was dismantled in New Hampshire, nettles spontaneously germinated in the composting horse manure. Europeans traditionally planted gardens and orchards in areas where nettles grew, using them as an indicator of good soil.

The Nova Scotia Department of Agriculture and Marketing warns tourists that nettles grow readily throughout the province in almost any soil and quickly form extensive colonies. However, rather than attempt to eradicate the nettles with herbicides, take advantage of your good fortune and utilize nettles for delightful dining and health care products.

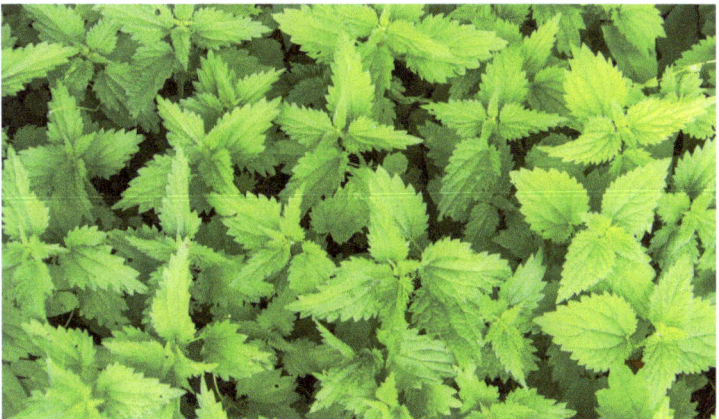

Harvesting: Keep it Safe, Keep it Legal

Harvest plants well away from all roads to avoid contamination from car exhaust, road salts, and pollutants. Avoid sprayed areas.

In the United States, you may freely harvest nettles in national forests provided that you remain 200 feet (61 meters) back from established trails, campgrounds, and roads.

Off limit to foragers are parks (state, national and municipal). On private lands, obtain permission before harvesting; locate owners via tax records at your local town hall or council office. A polite approach and small gifts of appreciation, such as Nesto (nettle pesto), can help ensure your ongoing harvesting privileges.

Tips and Tricks for Stingless Harvesting

A boy, stung by a Nettle, ran home crying, to get his mother to blow on the hurt and kiss it. "Son," said the boy's mother, when she had comforted him, "the next time you come near a Nettle, grasp it firmly, and it will be as soft as silk."

- The Boy and the Nettle, Aesop, 1919

Though I strongly advise those new to nettle harvesting or averse to the stings to wear gloves, I prefer direct contact between hands and herbs. I do take care to protect the sensitive skin between the wrist and elbows with a long-sleeved shirt. These areas of skin are especially susceptible and may form welts from nettle stings.

Before I begin to pick the tender tops, I follow the customs of my Mi'kmaq ancestors, asking permission from the nettles to harvest. I thank nettles for their gifts via a song, prayer, or token. (This ritual is intrinsic to diverse indigenous cultures throughout Alaska and the globe.)

After an enthusiastic harvesting session, my hands may 'tingle' for 24 to 48 hours. In my personal experience, this 'tingling' yields sustained therapeutic benefit. My right hand once had a marked tendency to become numb when exposed to damp cold. After

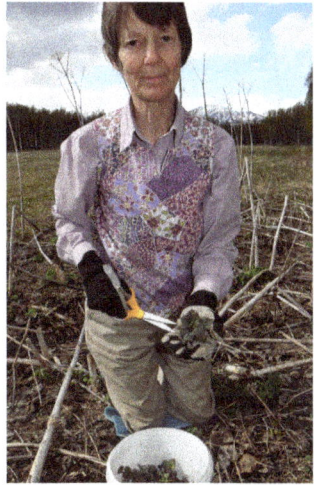

Ellen Vande Visse of Palmer, Alaska, is wearing gloves to harvest prime spring nettles.

seasons of nettle harvesting, it ceased troubling me, even when crossing Alaska's blustery Kachemak Bay in an open skiff in winter.

To minimize stinging, grasp the nettle firmly. Press the underside of nettle leaves against the stem. If you prefer to avoid being stung, simply wear a supple pair of gardening gloves. If you forget to bring them along, find a large non-toxic, non-thorny leaf and use it to wrap the nettle before snipping it with scissors or a knife.

There are many favorite ways to relieve nettle stings. You can follow the proverb: *"Nettle in, dock out."*

Need more options? Crush jewelweed leaves (*Impatiens noli-tangere*) or rub yourself with the brown chaff from young fiddlehead ferns. Or use aloe vera gel or a paste of baking soda and water.

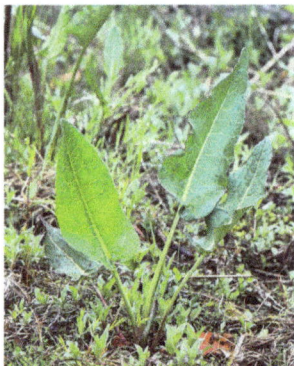

Rubbing nettle stings with crushed dock leaves (*Rumex* species) is a traditional remedy.

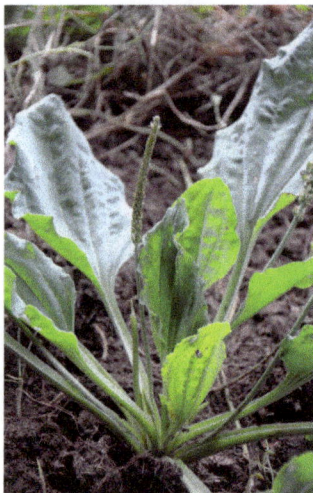

Plantain leaves (*Plantago major*) are a popular alternative.

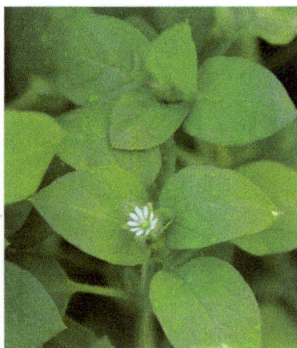

I also greatly favor the soothing properties of mashed chickweed (*Stellaria media*).

When to Harvest

Nettles are harbingers of spring. When the earth first begins to thaw, they emerge exuberantly from the cold soil. The ideal time for bulk harvesting is soon after emergence, when nettles are a few inches to a foot in height.

The primary spring nettle harvest in south-central Alaska generally concludes before the summer solstice. Indicators that they are 'past prime' include both the appearance of flowers, as well as flies or caterpillars that suddenly appear and plague the nettles, eating holes in their leaves. In Montana, aphids devour the older plants. Observation will reveal the signs specific to your local area. Look for insect infestation or a loss of vibrancy as shown by color change (paler in hue).

Industrious foragers can gather nettles into the summer. But limit harvest to the young growing tips and scattered young plants growing in their elders' shadow. Even when flowering, tender young growth exists at the top; pick and dry for tea or steamed as a vegetable.

Note that nettles, like mints, thrive on being picked. They branch readily and produce new growth. Henriette Kress of Helsinki, Finland, extends her harvest by taking her hoe to her nettle patch, which sparks new shoots. She advises doing this up to five times during the season.

Harvesting Seeds After Flowering

After leaves have passed their prime, harvest the thick drooping female nettle seed clusters. Herbal Ed Smith of HerbPharm recommends, "Don't wait too long for the seed to mature and let the calyx deteriorate. I find the seed/calyx to be very tasty and nourishing, and I recommend them, especially for hypothyroid conditions. Nettle seed is a popular folk cancer remedy in Turkey."

Dry the female seed clusters before eating (or storing). Hand-pick the thick green seed clusters from nettle plants and dry them in a dehydrator or in an oven on low heat. Alternately, cut the stalks, tie in bundles to dry.

Use the seeds/capsules in trail balls, green drinks, trail bars, hair products, and animal feed.

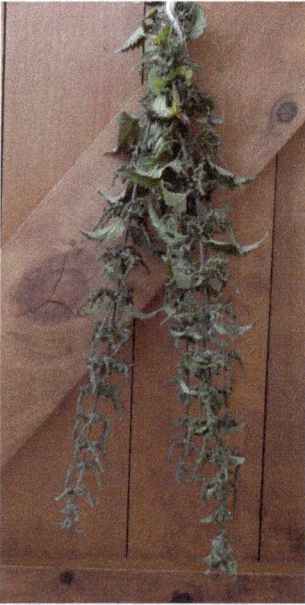

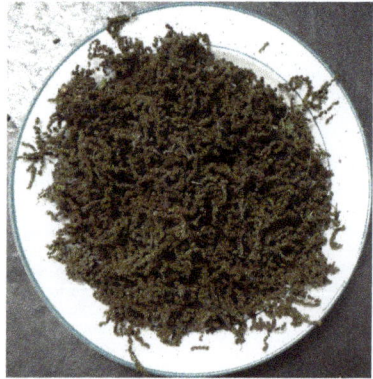

After drying, remove the seed/calyx, discarding the mature plant leaves.

Harvesting Roots

Autumn to early spring are the prime seasons to harvest roots for medicinal use. (I live in a snow-free area where I can dig roots even in the depth of winter.) Dig the trailing roots and wash well. A vegetable brush is excellent for removing clinging dirt.

Dangers: Nettle Species to Avoid

When hiking in the backcountry in New Zealand, and seeing its native nettle (*Urtica ferox*), I immediately knew I'd met a nettle that demanded extraordinary respect. The stinging hairs of this nettle are fierce.

Indeed, this 'tree nettle' (called *ongaonga* by Maori) is reputed to have killed animals who tumbled down slopes into its dense patches. And literature also recorded a human's death in 1961. This robust nettle can grow to 6 feet (2 meters) in height and has distinct white stinging hairs.

Tree nettle's stinging toxins may induce impaired breathing, profuse salivation, and potential death.[3]

If resident or visitor to India and Java, avoid its native *U. urentissima*. Stings from this devil's leaf nettle are described as hot branding irons on the skin. Equally unfriendly are the Asian species, *U. crenulato* and *U. heterophylla*. (Interestingly, India does also have an unusual nettle species with nutritious tubers, appropriately named *U. tuberosa*.)[4]

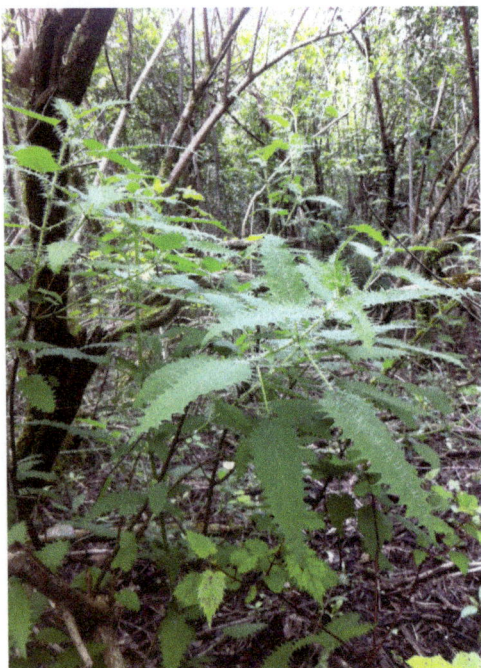

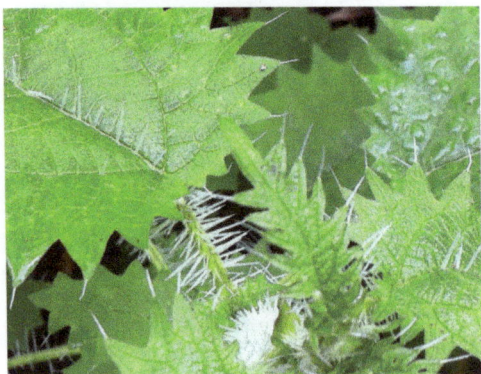

The fierce stinging hairs of
New Zealand's *Urtica ferox*.

Avoid Eating Old Nettles

Consuming the older leaves of mature nettle plants is discouraged. Not only do they become tough, gritty, and challenging to digest, they can potentially irritate the kidney. Irritation is due to crystal-like concretions called cystoliths (i.e., calcium carbonate deposits on the nettle's epidermal cells) in the mature plant. Older nettles may also contain phytoliths, sometimes called "plant opals." Australian naturopath Andrew Pengelly adds: "I've not heard of the kidney irritation theory, but I wouldn't discount it. Silicates remain undigested in the body and require excretion through the kidneys. Consumption of old nettle plants will increase the general gravel or inorganic sludge that our kidneys have to deal with."

Clinical herbalist Paul Bergner adds that two of his students had kidney irritation after drinking infusions of old nettles. The problem eased when they stopped the nettles. Bergner recommends asking companies that sell nettles, "when were they harvested?" He adds that "due to the inconsistency of product quality, I also think we should reconsider automatically saying that nettles are safe in pregnancy. It may depend on the proper harvesting of the plant."

Otherwise, ingesting young nettles in virtually any form (except the raw plant) is generally safe. As with any new food, proceed cautiously to ascertain that you are not one of the uncommon individuals with an allergy to nettles. Nettle leaf or seeds may, on rare occasions, cause gastrointestinal irritation, edema, or skin rashes. Contact urticaria–from unintentionally tangling with wild nettles–is by far the most common nettle-related malady.

A Strange Nettle Sport

Despite the recommendations above not to eat raw nettles, England's competitors do precisely that in an annual competition at the Bottle Inn in Dorset. The event evolved from a 'longest nettle' bet. When farmer Alix Williams won with his 15-foot, 6 inches (4.6 meters) nettle, he boasted that if anyone could beat his prize nettle, he'd eat it. A 16-foot nettle (4.8 meters) trumped his champion, and he made good on his bet.

Today, competitors worldwide gather into the Dorset World Nettle Eating Championships annually to vie for the distinction of being the person who consumes the most raw nettle leaves.

Mashing the raw plants between the fingers, as many competitors do, breaks down the stinging hairs (though heating or drying remains the most reliable method by far for safely eating nettles). In the Dorset competition, the leaves are from mature nettles. Though one may be 'fine' consuming them for a single day, I hold to the recommendation of consuming young nettles only.

Other Nettle Family Members

The nettle family, as a whole, comprises approximately 500 species divided into 54 genera. Family members vary from herbs and shrubs to trees and vines. Many lack stinging hairs.

An infamous Australian rainforest nettle family member is the stinging tree, gympie gympie (*Dendrocnide*). Its razor-sharp silica hairs trigger severe burning, which lasts for hours. Burning recurs when contacting cold water or experiencing temperature fluctuations. The alternating burning, and temporary relief, can endure for months and, in some cases, has led to an agonising death.

A far more friendly nettle is pellitory of the wall (*Parietaria officinalis*) traditionally used for urinary complaints and wound ointments. *Boehmeria* or false nettle, a stingless family member, is grown in the southern United States as an ornamental. Asians cultivate *B. nivea* (ramie) for fiber. Various species of *Pilea*, another stingless nettle, are often grown ornamentally for hanging baskets. The artillery plant, *P. microphylla*, is so named for its habit of forcibly ejecting pollen from the floral anthers.[5]

Some plants in other families with 'nettle' names, for example, hedge nettle (*Stachys*), hemp nettle (*Galeopsis*), and dead nettle (*Lamium*) are, in actuality, mints. And bull nettle (*Cnidoscolus*) is a spurge.

Readers Notes

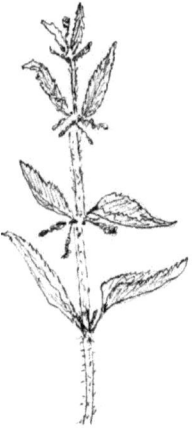

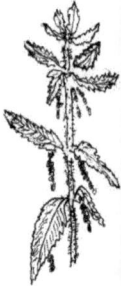

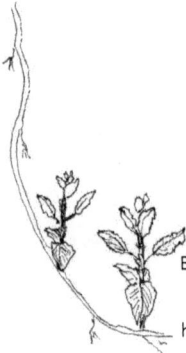

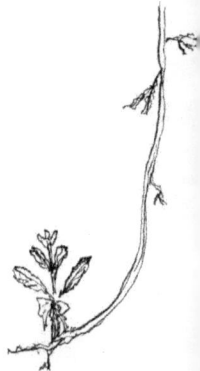

E-mail your new recipes and nettle experiences to:
athomewithjanice@gmail.com
for potential inclusion in the blog:
https://www.athomewithjaniceschofieldeaton.com

Chapter 2

Nettles In The Kitchen

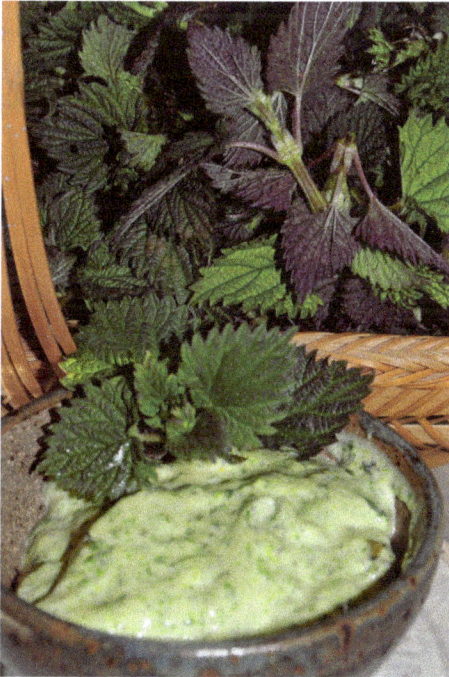

"To Mr. Symons, where we found him abroad, but she, like a good lady, within and there we did eat some nettle porridge, which was made on purpose today for some of their coming, and was very good."

- Diary of Samuel Pepys, February 1661

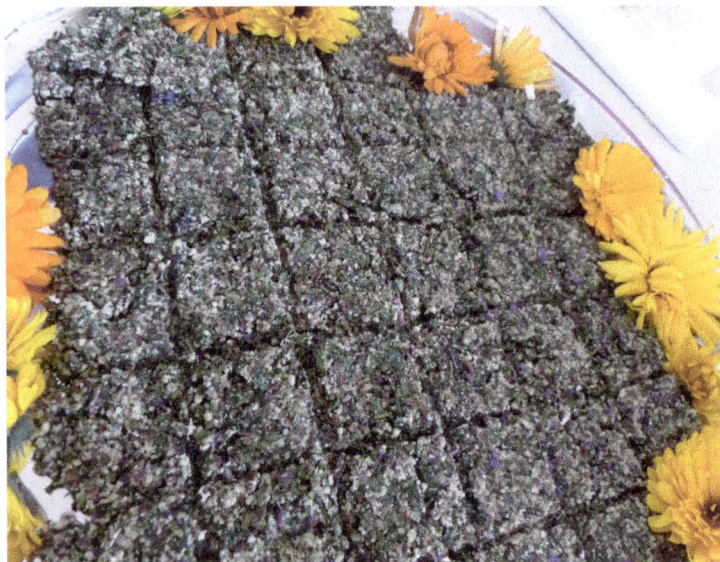

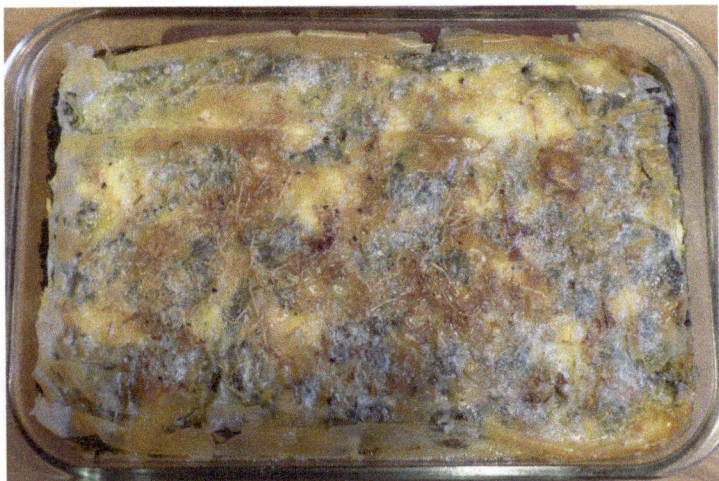

Fresh Nettles

From ancient times to techno times, nettles have received kudos for culinary adaptability. They are a prime example of 'food as medicine.' Adding nettles to one's cuisine adds gourmet flavor and a wide variety of nutrients.

Novices wonder how one can eat a plant that stings the skin. The answer lies in steaming or boiling the herb. Either method tames the nettle and renders it palatable for consumption. (Drying also deactivates stings.)

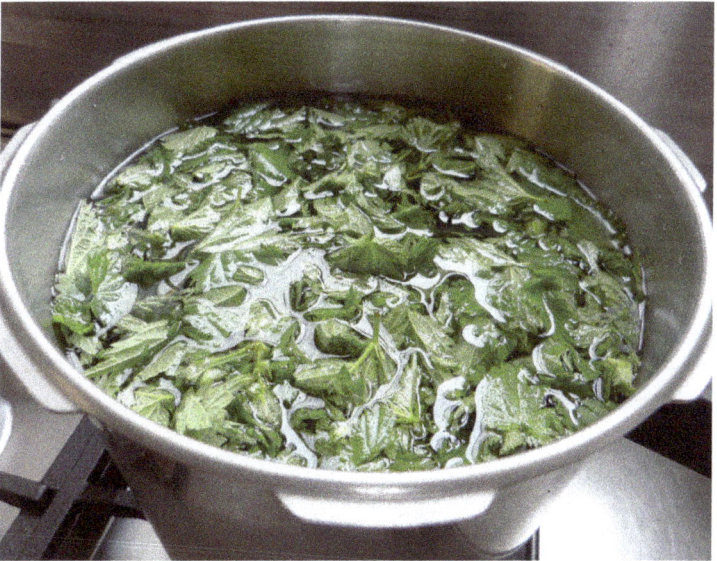

Nettles are not recommended raw as a salad green–unless you have access to the Hungarian *U. galeopsifolia* (sometimes classed as *U. dioica* subspecies *galeopsifolia*) which truly is stingless.

A student assured me that Alaska's nettles *Urtica Lyallii* and *U. gracilis* have a stingless phase. She nibbled them raw, she claimed, in early spring when first peeking from the earth. When I attempted to duplicate her feat, I promptly received a tingling 'nettle lip.' Another student's tip was: twist shoots between gloved or calloused fingers to thoroughly crush the stinging hairs. A friend who attempted this trick, and consumed the nettles, received nettle stings in her throat.

The latest tip I've heard is to FIRMLY stroke the nettle to crush the hairs and then roll the mass into a ball. (This technique is practiced by a number of participants in the annual British raw nettle-eating contest). I prefer safety over drunken feats, and recommend fresh young nettles in cooked dishes. Heat is a definite way to deactivate their sting.

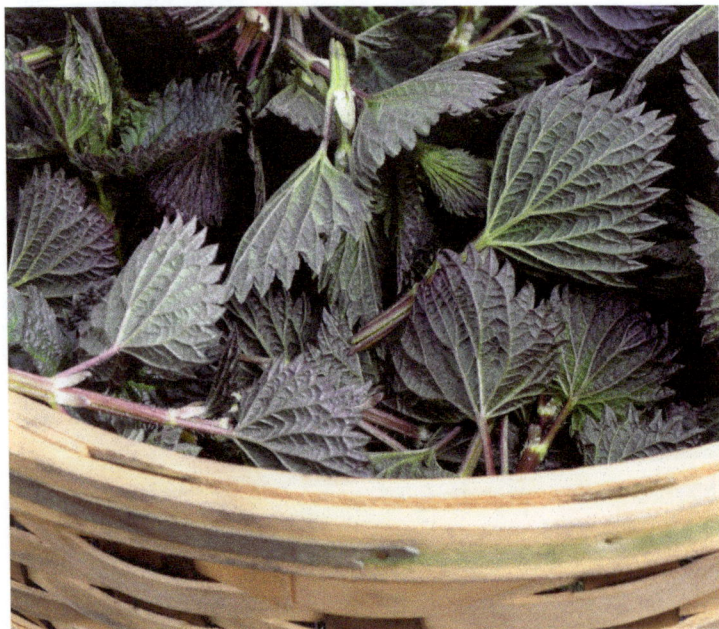

Gather nettles in pristine areas, well away from roads and dust. Pinch or snip the young tips; avoid uprooting any plants. Collect the top 3 to 4 inches. Plants 6-8 inches high are ideal. To encourage the plant to sprout new shoots, snip just above a pair of leaves. On taller young plants gather the upper portion that is still close together. Once plants start to flower, collect only the newly emerging leaves at the top.

Nettle Potherb

The word potherb dates back to 1538 and simply refers to leafy greens, like nettles, that are steamed or boiled as a vegetable.

Nettles are a traditional potherb in the rural districts of Great Britain and many other countries. They are typically cooked like spinach, swiss chard (silverbeet), collards, and other leafy greens.

Some authors insist that nettles need to be boiled for 10-15 minutes; I consider that total overkill. Nettles are rendered stingless as soon as they wilt: about 2-3 minutes. If steaming a large pot of nettles, rotate the layers by stirring to expose all to heat; otherwise, the innermost nettles may still be armed with stinging hairs.

If boiling a potful, you only need 1-2 inches of water in the bottom. Save the nutritious cooking water as a stock for soups and stews. (Or feed the cooled water to your plants or pets.) At an Alaskan Native elder gathering, I served nettle pesto on crackers and small cups of nettle cooking water as taste-testers during my pre-luncheon talk.

Serve the cooked nettle greens 'as is,' or enhanced with olive oil, a touch of butter, ghee (clarified butter), a sprinkling of Parmesan, or your favorite topping.

Herbalist Rosemary Gladstar, the founder of the California School of Herbal Studies, Traditional Medicinal Tea, and SAGE, describes nettles as: ". . . absolutely my favorite herb. I'm thoroughly addicted to the taste and would trade the best pint of ice cream in the world for a bowl of fresh steamed nettle greens sprinkled with Feta cheese, olive oil, and a dab of lemon."

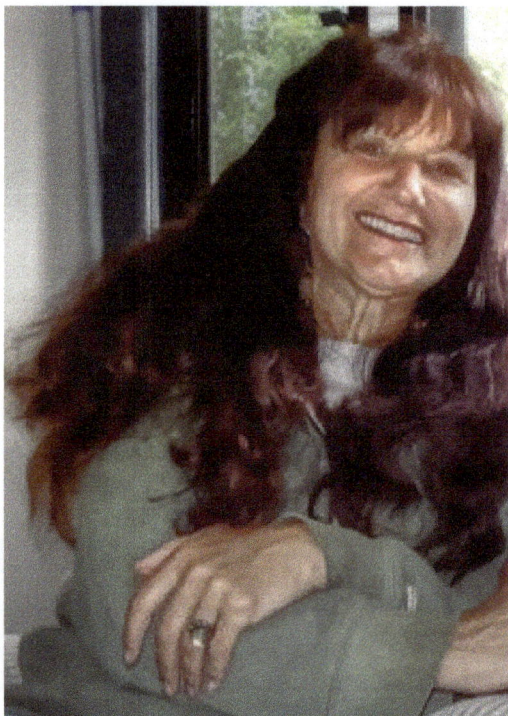

My herbal mentor, Rosemary Gladstar

Noko's Nettles

a Japanese-style nettle potherb
by Noko Yoshida, Homer, Alaska

Boil nettles (as much as desired) and blanch quickly in cold water. Top with a blend of:

3 tablespoons rice vinegar

1 1/2 teaspoons sugar

3 tablespoons dashi (Japanese soup stock)

dash of soy sauce

In my Noko's Nettles taste test, I substituted honey in place of sugar.

You can buy dashi at an Asian supermarket or make it yourself with kombu sea vegetables and dried fish flakes (traditionally bonito) steeped in water. (Abundant dashi recipes are on the internet.)

Saving Nettles For Year-round Use

Freezing: To blanch or not to blanch?

Blanching is the most traditional method for preserving nettles for extended culinary nettle use. Chop nettles to a manageable size. Have two pots available, one with boiling water, one with cold. Plunge coarsely chopped greens in rapidly boiling water for 1-2 minutes. Strain, and quickly plunge in cold water for 2 minutes. Strain well. Place in freezer.

Or, to save time in the kitchen and preserve nutrients, snip unblanched nettles directly into a resealable plastic bag (or glass jar) and freeze. Try both methods and see which you prefer.

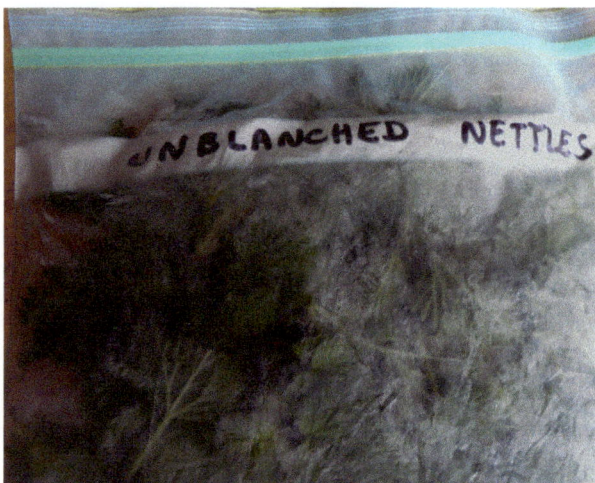

Another option is to prepare nettle pesto (following) and freeze the pesto in small jars or ice cube trays. I generally freeze two to three dozen jars of "Nesto" annually.

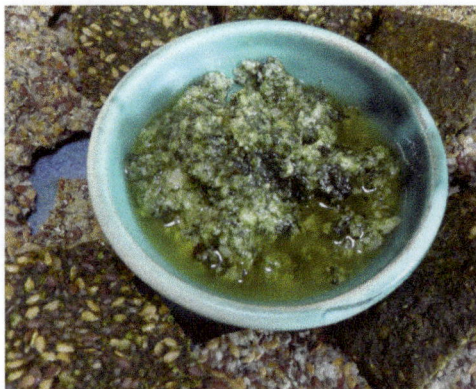

Nesto (Nettle Pesto)

This recipe is highly flexible and varies depending on my mood, available ingredients, and the number of nettles available. Below is a guideline to get you started:

4 cups steamed, boiled, or sauteed nettles

3-6 cloves garlic, finely minced or pressed

1/4-1/3 cup finely grated Parmesan cheese (dairy or vegan)

freshly squeezed juice from 1-2 lemons

4-6 tablespoons pine nuts, sunflower seeds, cashews or other nuts of choice

1/2 teaspoon sea salt or Celtic salt

1/4-1/3 cup extra virgin olive oil (add more or less oil as desired)

Cool nettles and then squeeze well to remove excess water (save the juice for soups). Then place all ingredients in a food processor. (If using a blender, chop cooked nettles before adding; you also may wish to pre-grind the nuts or seeds.) Whiz well to a paste. Adjust the amount of olive oil and lemon juice for the perfect consistency for your needs.

Use thicker Nesto for pasta or pizza sauce, dips, and sandwich spreads. For salad dressing, thin with extra olive oil and lemon juice.

Nesto Variations

Try adding sun-dried tomatoes, kalamata olives, cilantro, or basil to Nesto for extra flavor.

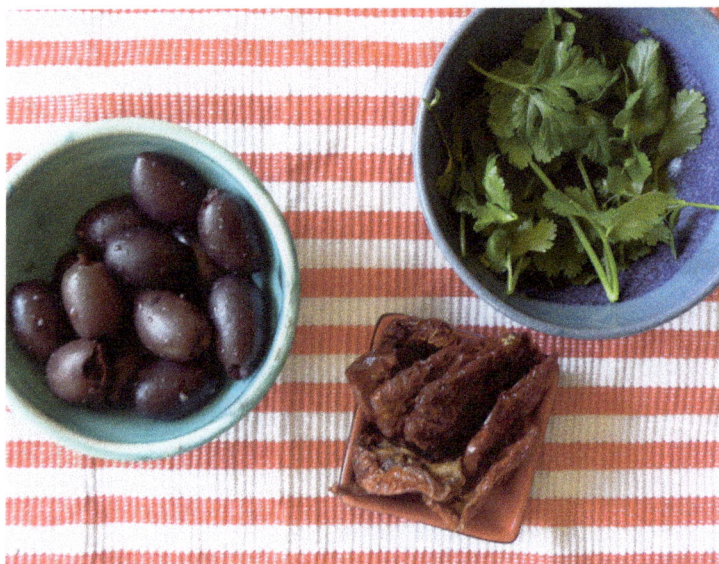

Nesto (raw version)

The idea of making nettle pesto with the young uncooked greens was introduced to me by Vidhi Marshall of Rangiora, New Zealand. Vidhi described the raw pesto she had made as 'incredibly delicious.' As you know, I am dubious about consuming raw nettles, even if mashed or pureed. And Vidhi confessed that one batch she'd made left a 'stinging sensation' in her mouth. We pondered how to reap the superior flavor while reliably avoiding an undesirable sting.

The solution (which thus far has worked 100 percent) was inspired by Vidhi's goat Corinna.

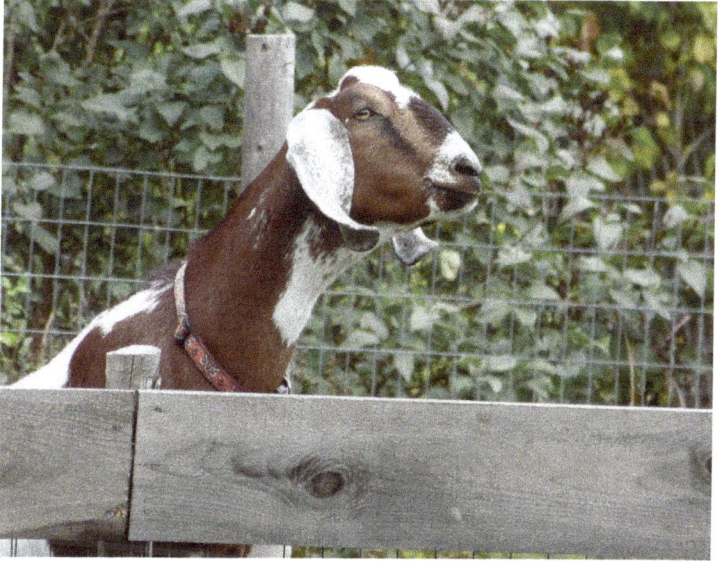

Vidhi noticed that the wise nanny avoided nettles except on frosty days. Using myself as a guinea pig, I froze bowls of raw nettles. I then toasted cashews in a skillet and pureed them with frozen nettles, extra virgin olive oil, lemon juice, grated Parmesan, and a bit of Celtic Salt. The pesto was fabulous.

Preservation: Nettle pesto freezes beautifully. Make repeated batches in season and freeze in 1/2 pint jars. Nesto is a scrumptious hors d'oeuvre for potlucks or unexpected company or a special treat for the whole family.

Whichever Nesto recipe you prefer, try serving the result with the following Nettle Crackers.

Nettle Crackers

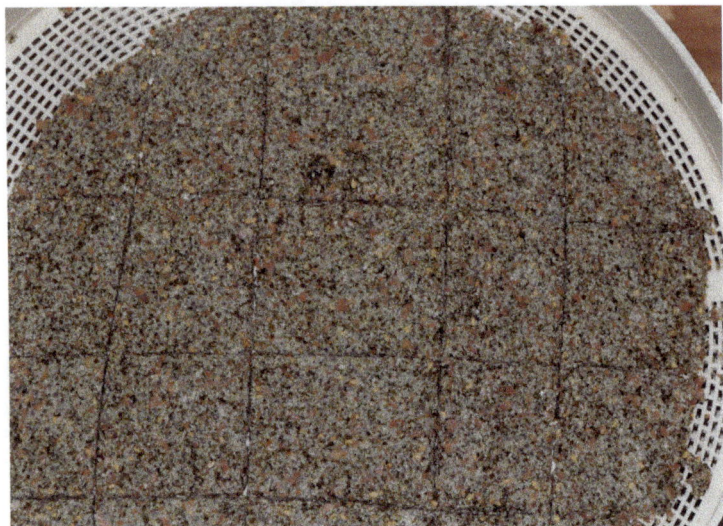

These crackers are an economical alternative to the gluten-free crackers sold in shops. They are ideal for low-carbohydrate diets and a fabulous way to use ground nuts or seeds leftover from making dairy-free milk.

Note: When making nut or seed milk, save your drained nuts and freeze. Make crackers when you've accumulated enough for a batch.

Gluten-free Nettle Crackers

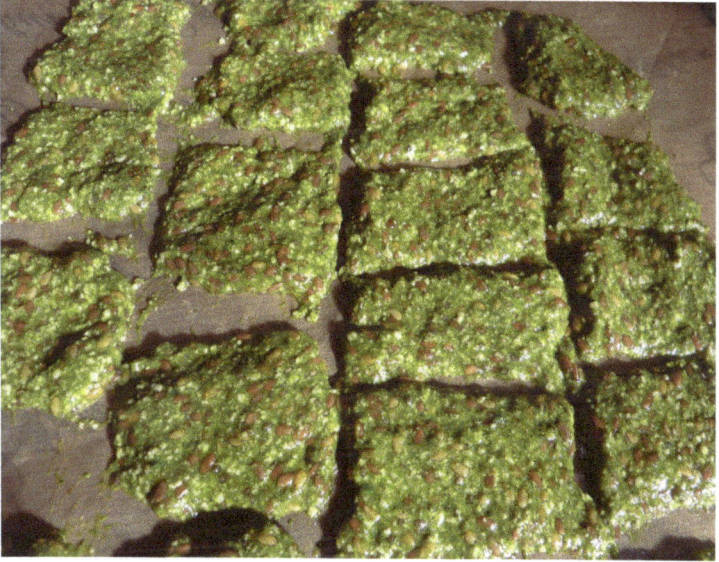

Have ready:

>1 cup Nesto (previous recipe)

>In jar or bowl, combine:

>1 cup cashews

>1 cup flax seed

>¼ cup chia seed

>3 cups water

Soak the above ingredients for at least 2 hours (or overnight). Drain, discarding the soak water. Add 3 cups of freshwater. Whiz well. Drain, saving the ground seeds and cashews.

In a bowl, combine ingredients. The cracker dough will be quite 'gooey.' Spread thinly onto silicon sheets, scoring into crackers shapes, before putting trays into a dehydrator or oven on a low setting. (In my home, I have an Excalibur dehydrator that I set at 125 degrees F. (50 degrees C.) and heat 6-8 hours or until crispy. Halfway through the drying process, I flip the crackers over onto the screen and remove the silicon sheet.) Drying time will vary according to the method used. Makes 3 to 4 dozen small crackers.

Cracker Variations

Vary the types of nuts and seeds. Add gluten-free flour if desired. Instead of pesto, use pureed steamed nettles or rehydrated dry nettles. Add sundried tomato or olives. Try with mashed pumpkin and spices like cumin and garlic. Add roasted onion or other herbs.

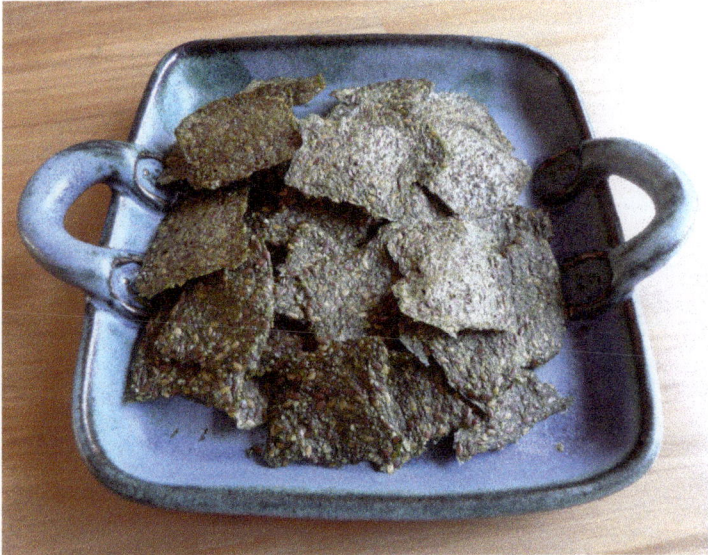

An easy recipe for Nut or Seed Milk

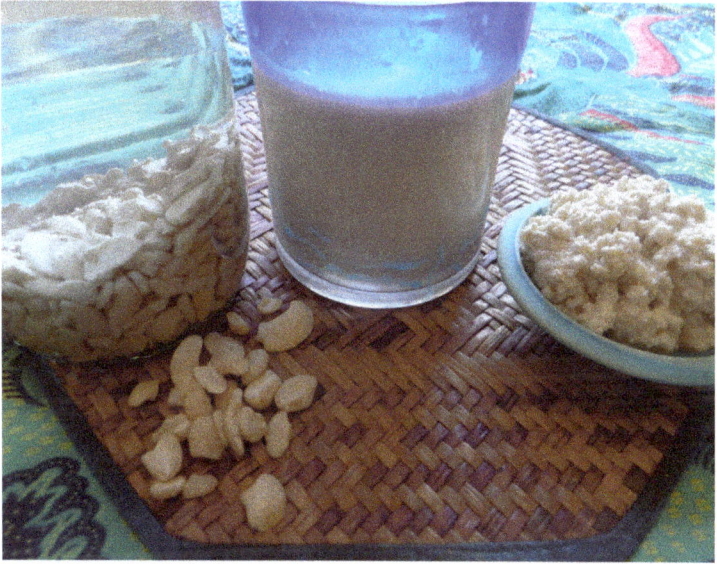

Almond milk, cashew milk, walnut milk, sunflower seed milk, etc., are expensive to buy yet simple to make. Place 1 cup nuts or seeds of choice in a jar and cover with 5 cups water. Let sit overnight. In the morning, drain and discard the water.

To the drained nuts, add fresh water and whiz in a blender, Vitamix, or 'bullet' type machine. How much water to add is a matter of choice. For a nut or seed 'cream' (to drizzle on a dessert or splash in coffee), use a ratio of 2:1, i.e., 2 cups water to 1 cup nuts or seeds. For nut milk, 4:1 is the standard ratio in online recipes. Due to the high cost of organic nuts, and my personal preferences, I tend to use 8:1 (8 cups water to 1 cup seeds or nuts). I find this more diluted nut milk more similar to a store-bought product. The 8:1 ratio is adequate for my general use, and it halves the cost of the end product.

Strain your whizzed creation. Use the milk in any recipe in place of dairy. To make your nut milk more 'fancy,' add a dollop of honey and a sprinkle of cinnamon, nutmeg, or cloves.

Save the ground drained nuts or seeds for use in cereal, desserts, or, of course, in these crackers. Soaking removes phytates–substances that keep nuts and seeds from prematurely germinating. Phytates are hard for our body to digest. Soaking (and disposing of the soak water) enhances digestibility.

Nettle Pizza

Buy or prepare a pizza crust. Top with Nesto and your favorite toppings, such as fresh mushrooms, roasted peppers, feta cheese, olives, artichoke hearts, capers, etc. Bake at 375 degrees F. (190 C.) for 20 minutes or as directed for your particular pizza crust.

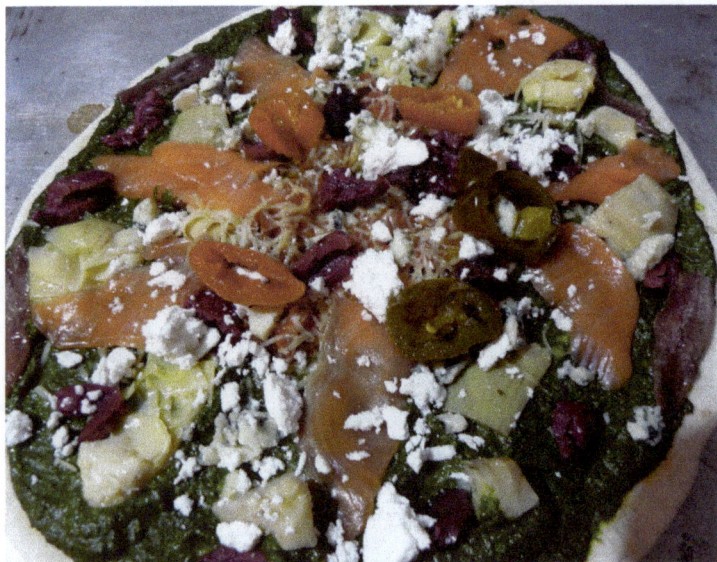

Stacy Studebaker of Kodiak, Alaska, makes a bodacious wild pizza using a wholewheat crust topped with nettle pesto, lady fern fiddleheads, fireweed shoots, beach lovage, smoked salmon, mozzarella cheese, and pine nuts. Check out her photo-illustrated step-by-step instructions on her website: https://senseofplacepress.com.

Nettle Soups

California herbalist and Reiki master Marina Bokelman views nettles as her secret ingredient in any soup, stew, or bean dish. "Whenever I can get away with adding a handful of crushed nettle, I do," says Marina.

Nettle soups are famous throughout the world. Tasmanian hostel operator Julia Weston often prepares her mother's favorite chicken stock enriched with potatoes, onions, and nettles. Nässelsoppa is a traditional Swedish recipe featuring nettles simmered with potatoes and chives, then pureed and mixed with cream.

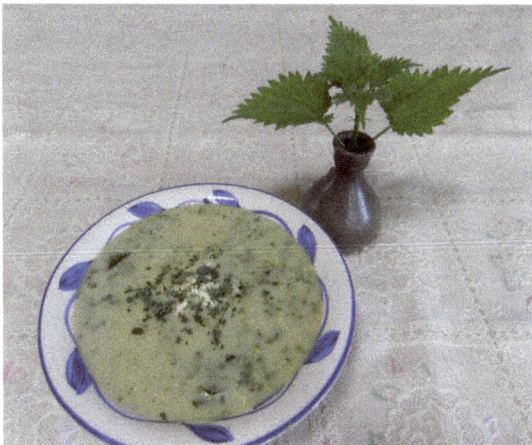

Nettle chowder is a family favorite of mine, a blend of onion, celery, mushrooms, corn, carrots, potatoes, nettles, salmon, nettle broth, milk (or nut milk), and spices.

Tips for Sensational Soups and Broths

1. Save water from cooking nettles for soup stock.

2. Add sundried tomatoes to nettle broth for extra flavor (great for a soup base, cooking rice, or enjoying a hot brew.

3. Simmer nettles with bones for an herbal bone broth.

4. Freeze nettle broth varieties in ice cube trays. Add cubes to casseroles or stir-fries for extra flavor and nutrition.

Laura Krieger's Spring Cleansing Soup

2 medium onions, sliced

1 medium beet, julienned or grated

1 carrot, thin-sliced

2 garlic cloves, thinly sliced

2 cups nettles, chopped

1 tablespoon olive oil

1 cup parsley, chopped

salt and pepper, to taste

1 cup wild greens (dandelion, lamb's quarter, miner's lettuce, etc.)

1/2 cup fresh mushrooms (shitake, if possible), chopped

Sauté onions, beet, carrot, garlic cloves, nettle leaves, and wild greens in olive oil over very low heat until golden and limp. Add chopped parsley and 6 cups water or broth.

Simmer covered for 45 minutes to an hour. Season to taste.

This soup has infinite variations. Add wild spring beauty, miner's lettuce or spring fiddleheads, or whatever is available from the spring garden or root cellar. In the soup shown in the photo, I've added pumpkin and parsnip that had wintered over. For a very cleansing soup for the liver, add burdock root and dandelion root. Modify throughout the seasons for a year-round soup. Use dry nettles or frozen pesto when fresh is not available.

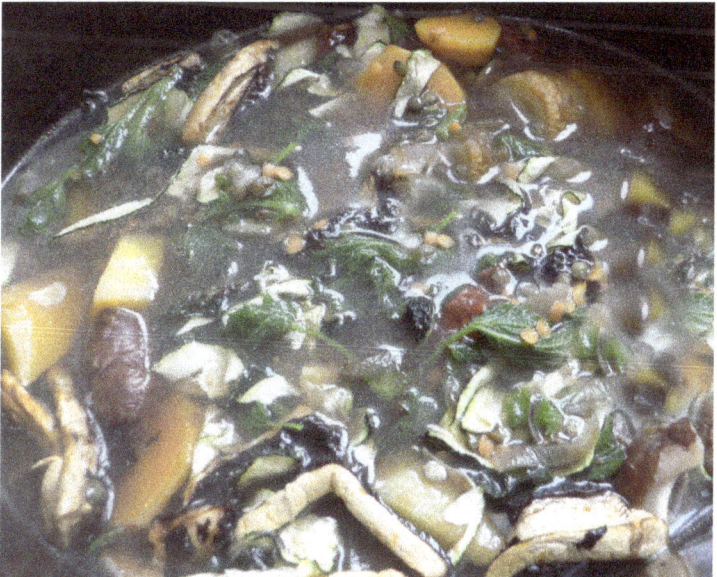

Nettles From Around The World

The popularity of nettles extends far beyond North American shores. Nettles are a perennial favorite from Tasmania to Turkey. In the latter country, nettles are often blended with sautéed minced meat and topped with yogurt.

Fussy children?

If you are introducing nettles to picky children or a fussy spouse, try the ideas from Italy. Kids of all ages love pasta. Add a Nesto layer in lasagna or atop a homemade pizza. Imitate Andreas Ryser's Swiss mother, and blend nettles with the more familiar garden spinach to surreptitiously add nutrition to family diets. Italian cuisine is a great starting point for around-the-world kitchen adventures.

Note: Those on low carbohydrate diets can substitute zoodles (spiralized zucchini) or kelp noodles instead of wheat noodles. The gluten-sensitive also have abundant noodle options, including sweet potato, black bean, rice, and edame.

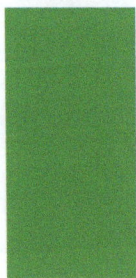

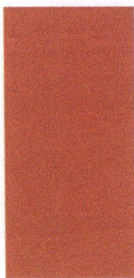

Nettles are fabulous in lasagna. Layer steamed nettles between the noodles. (Those on low-carb diets can use thin zucchini slices instead of noodles). If combined with abundant sauce, nettles can 'tame' themselves as they bake. I often use Nesto as a layer between the pasta sheets.

Fill homemade ravioli with nettles or Nesto. I especially like a filling of nettle-olive tapenade. An easy supper is penne pasta with cherry tomatoes, olive oil, chives, and finely chopped steamed nettles.

I first fell in love with Nettle Linguini in a University of Alaska plant lore class. Students Sonja Tobiessen and Mary Bee Kaufman created an exquisite dish. The following similar recipe was the product of Meadow Bejaro and Cordova, Alaska herb students.

Nettle Linguini

2 cups semolina flour

2 eggs

1-ounce extra-virgin olive oil

2 cups fresh Nettles (or 4 tablespoons dried, powdered nettles)

Steam fresh nettles. Drain well and chop fine. In a bowl, blend flour with eggs and oil. Knead in nettles. The dough should be pliable and able to be rolled. If too dry, add extra oil, a little at a time. Cover the dough with plastic wrap and allow it to rest for 15 minutes.

Roll dough thinly on a lightly floured board and cut into long strips, 1/4 inch (6 mm) wide (or use a pasta machine, following

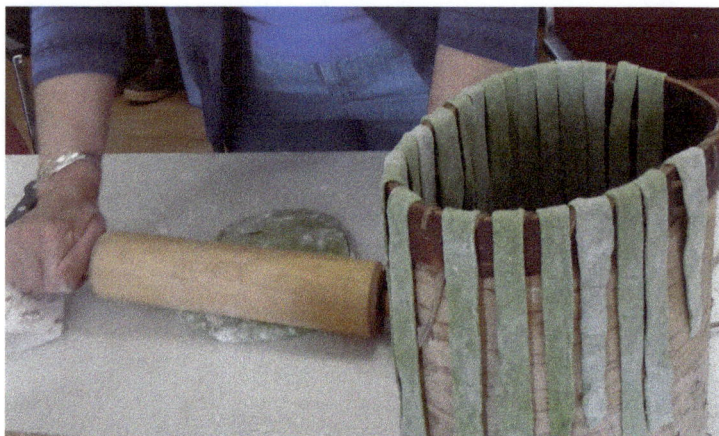

standard directions). Dry noodles lightly by hanging on the back of a chair draped with clean dishcloths.

Bring a large pot of water to a rapid boil. Add noodles, stirring with a fork to prevent clumping. Do not overcook. Test after two minutes for doneness. Serve with Nesto, white sauce, tomato sauce, or garlic/herb butter.

GREECE

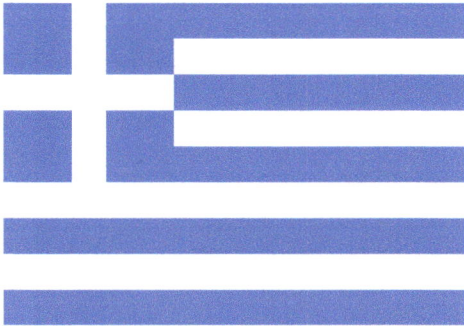

Greek Style Nettle Salad

Horiatiki is the 'classic' Greek salad featuring only tomato, cucumber, red onions, olives, green pepper, and Feta, seasoned with olive oil, vinegar, salt, and oregano. My variation features, of course, freshly steamed nettles.

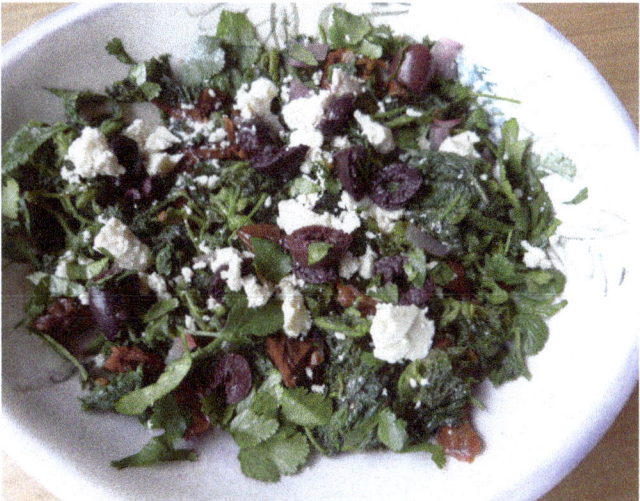

Nettles: 6-8 cups of steamed, drained nettles. Cool and coarsely chop.

Then drizzle with a marinade of your choice. My favorite is:

1 tablespoon vinegar (rice, apple cider, or balsamic)

1/3 cup extra-virgin olive oil

3-6 cloves garlic, pressed or finely minced

1 tablespoon lemon juice (more as desired)

salt and pepper

Marinate 2-4 hours or until ready to serve. Then garnish with your choice of 'classic' ingredients (Feta, cucumber, etc.)

Spanakopita

Rosemary Gladstar and the California School of Herbal Studies introduced me to a wild herb spanakopita four decades ago, and I've been making it ever since. Traditional spanakopita is a Greek spinach pie. Greens layer between thin sheets of filo (aka phyllo); this unleavened dough is readily available in supermarkets. Spanakopita is excellent served hot or cold. The dish is fabulous to take along on car or camping outings.

You will need a large potful of nettles: Steam or boil for 5 minutes. Then drain and set aside.

Other filling ingredients:

1 large, diced red onion

2 stalks, chopped celery

1 chopped capsicum:

1 teaspoon olive oil

Sauté above vegetables in olive oil until golden.

While heating the vegetables, spread 4 folded filo dough sheets in a pre-greased rectangular baking dish (13.5-inch x 8 inch; 340mm x 200mm;).

Blend the nettles with the cooked vegetables. Chop well. Spread the chopped steamed, drained nettle and vegetable mixture over the filo.

In a separate bowl, mix:

1/2 package of Feta cheese

6-8 eggs, beaten

1/4 cup milk or nut milk

salt, pepper, and seasonings to taste.

Pour the cheese-egg mixture over the filling. Cover with 4 (or more if desired) sheets of folded filo dough. Place pats of butter or drops of olive oil on top. Bake at 200 C. (375 F.) for 30 minutes or until golden.

This recipe is endlessly adaptable and expandable. The pastry becomes flaky when baked. Now that I am doing a low-carb lifestyle, I found myself missing filo. I've happily discovered I can make my own with coconut-flour/psyllium seed instead of wheat! (Check the internet for grain-free filo recipes.)

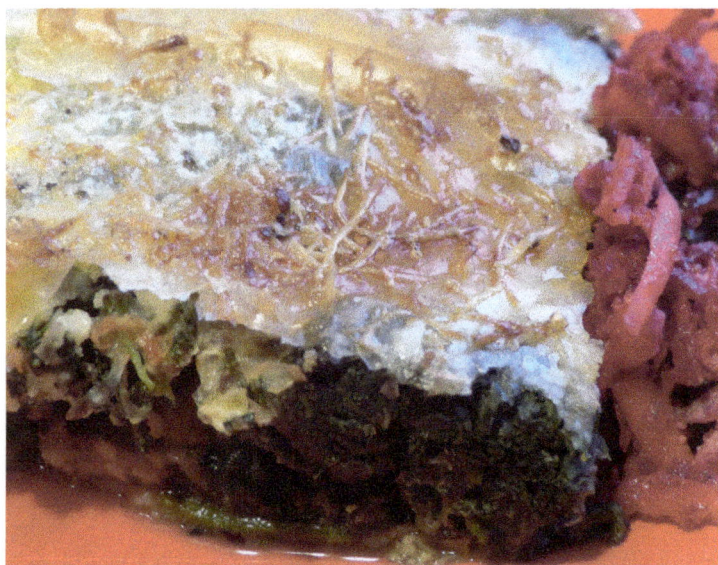

Nettle-based Spanakopita

FRANCE

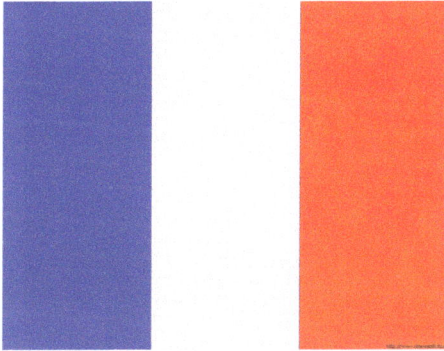

Tourte Saordienne

Tourtes are savory pies, typically featuring spring greens. Nettle-rich tourtes, like the following one taught to me by French visitor Marie Noelle Pignolet, are classic throughout rural France.

Crust:

2 1/2 cups (400 g) flour

1/3 cup water plus 1 Tb. +/-

1 teaspoon salt

3/4 cup olive oil

Filling:

> about 4 cups total: spring nettles, silverbeet (Swiss chard), plus a lesser quantity of thyme, borage, oregano
>
> 1 onion, diced
>
> 2 eggs, beaten
>
> 1/4 cup olive oil
>
> 1/2 tsp. salt and pepper

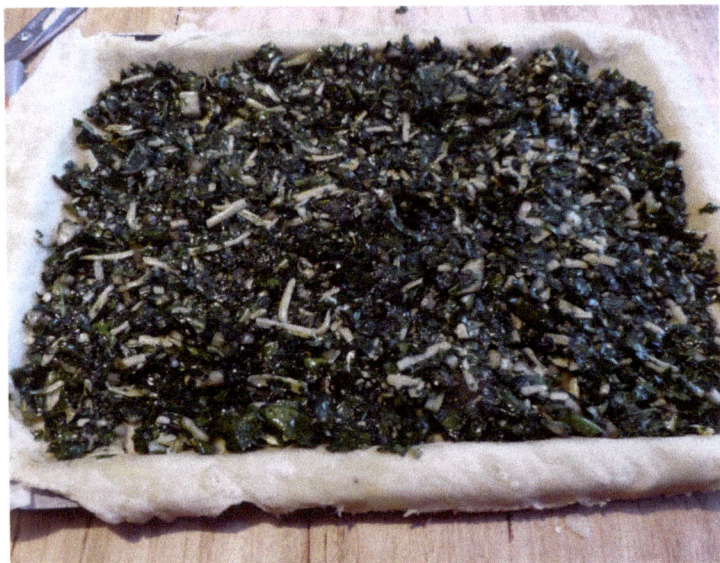

Preheat oven 375-400 degrees F. (180-200 degrees C.). Prepare the dough by mixing the flour, water, olive oil, and salt. The dough should be soft, not elastic.

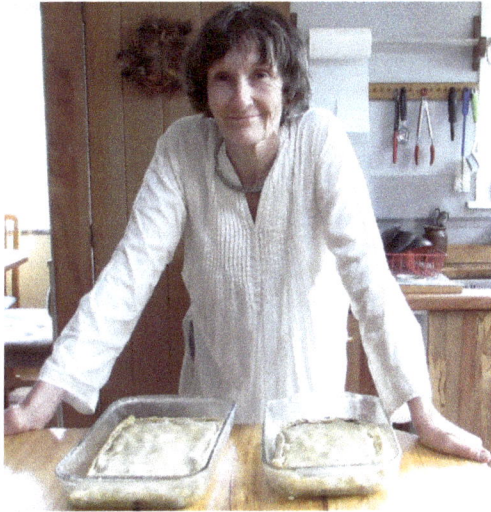

Marie Noelle Pignolet ready to bake the nettle tourte

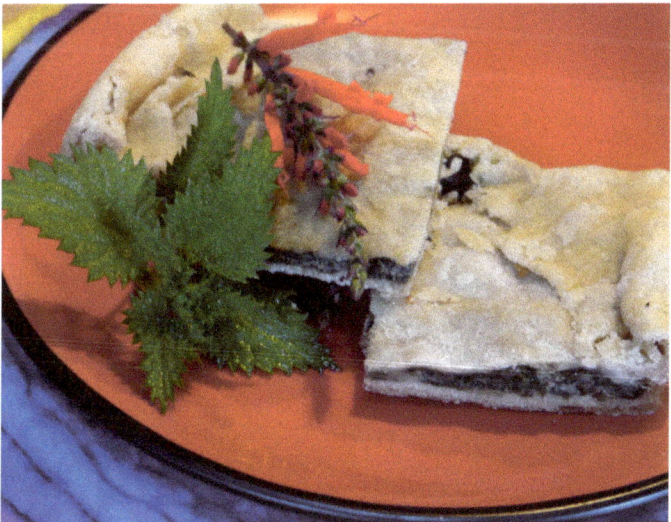

Marie cautions: "Do not overwork the dough. Lift the dough gently as you mix the ingredients." Add water in slowly and gently shape, using very light pressure.

While the dough is resting (15 minutes), blend beaten eggs, greens, seasonings, and oil in a separate bowl. Then divide the dough into 2 balls, one a bit larger than the other. Roll each ball out on a floured board as thinly as possible. Use the larger dough for the bottom crust; place in a greased pie plate. Fill with the vegetable mixture.

Cover with the top crust. Pinch the edges together around the rim.

Bake in a hot oven for about 20 minutes. Do not overcook (as it would dry out the pie.)

BRITAIN

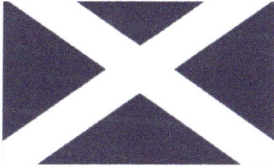

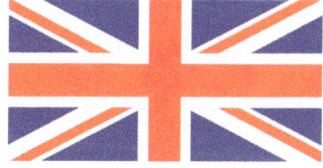

Flags of Scotland and Britain

Nettle Haggis

"But mark the Rustic, haggis fed,
The trembling earth resounds his tread."

– Robert Burns, "Address to a Haggis"

Though Scots celebrate haggis as their national dish and 'pipe in' the haggis (with bagpipes), Brits insist that haggis is Britain's oldest recipe, dating from 6000 B.C. Haggis appears in Scottish and British herbals with many variations. Haggis recipes typically include nettles, oatmeal or barley, onions, spices, and ground sheep heart, liver, and lungs, slowly simmered in a sheep stomach. Though the idea of eating offal sounds awful to many moderns, haggis (when properly prepared) is a nutrient-dense dish and highly revered for its flavor.

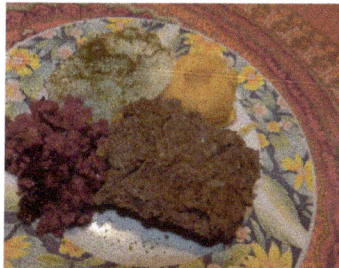

The haggis shown here is a traditional lamb-offal blend given to me by a New Zealander of Scottish descent. The specific recipe, however, remained a closely guarded secret.

The Scottish Federation of Meat Traders hosts an annual Haggis championship.

Vegetarian Nettle Haggis

4 cups fresh nettles, chopped

3 cloves garlic, minced

1 leek, chopped

1 cup oatmeal

2 tablespoons olive oil

1 teaspoon each sage, thyme, salt, pepper

Sauté all ingredients in a large frypan until greens wilt. Place in a bowl, and let cool. Then press the mixture into a ball.

Place in a jelly bag; Simmer 45 minutes in water or vegetable stock. Serve with your choice of toppings, such as gravy or Nesto.

FINLAND

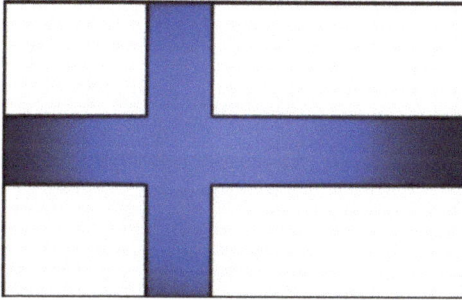

From Finland comes the recipe of herbalist Henriette Kress. Like me, Henriette tends to cook with a dab of this and a dollop of that. The following recipe reflects that style.

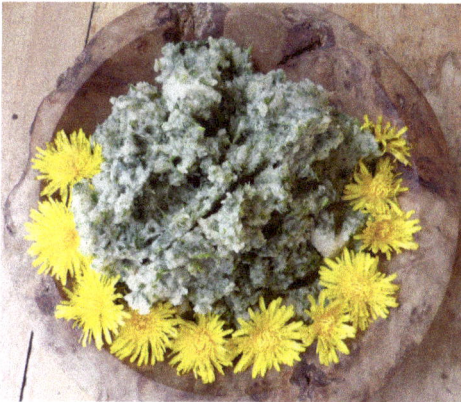

Henriette's Potato Mash

The amount of potatoes and nettles will depend on the size of your family. Be bold and experiment! In my taste test, I used 5 medium potatoes and 4 cups of fresh nettles.

Cook peeled potatoes with a bit of salt, beat them to a pulp, add some milk (or the cooking water) and butter or ghee. Add spices of choice (salt, pepper, nutmeg or mace, parsley or lovage, to taste). Add pre-cut, preboiled nettles. Stir together well and serve.

Another variation is to make potato patties. To the mash, add beaten eggs and a bit of flour. Panfry until golden in a bit of oil.

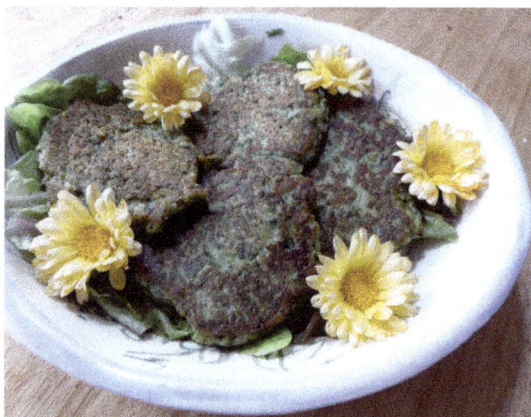

"This goes well with onions, fried until golden brown," comments Henriette, " and perhaps some carrots, green beans, green peas or corn topped with butter and a dash of salt."

I also like adding Parmesan or sun-dried tomatoes.

EASTERN EUROPE

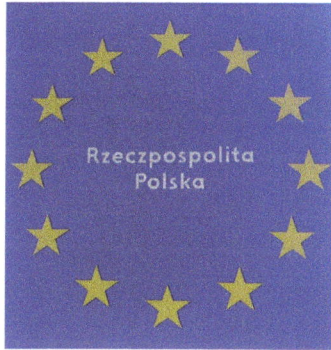

Flag of Poland

Popular at Easter in Czech culture is nádivka (aka hlavička), a salty cake made from bread soaked in milk, with eggs, spices, and spring nettles. In Prague, a restaurant offered ice cream made with nettles, pears, and radish.

In Poland, you can find Pokrzywianka, a creamy stinging nettle soup. On the north coast of Poland, a nettle crayfish soup features in its cuisine.

MEXICO

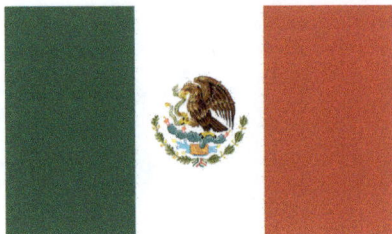

Ginny Moore's Nettle Quesadillas

This Mexican-style recipe is sure to please the family.

12 corn tortillas

Filling:

8 cups fresh nettle greens, chopped

1 tablespoon olive oil

1 medium onion, chopped

1 garlic clove, minced

1 pound fresh mushrooms, sliced

1 small can diced green chili

1 cup nettle cooking water

1-2 tablespoons fresh cilantro, chopped

salt and pepper, to taste

1 cup cheddar cheese, grated

1 cup Jack cheese, shredded

Garnish: salsa of choice

Steam nettles and set aside, reserving cooking water. Heat olive oil in a medium non-stick skillet on medium-high heat; add onion and cook for 3 to 5 minutes until softened. Add garlic and mushrooms and cook, stirring often, until mushrooms are lightly browned (5 to 7 minutes). Add steamed, drained nettles, cilantro, chili peppers, and nettle water, and cook just long enough to heat thoroughly. Add salt and pepper to taste. Remove from the burner, but keep warm.

Lightly butter tortillas; heat in a skillet over medium-high heat for 30 seconds. Add filling to cover one-half of the tortilla; then top it with cheese mixture. Fold tortilla in half and lightly brown both sides, 30 seconds on each side. Serve with salsa. Serves four.

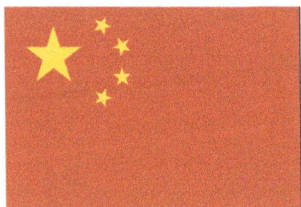

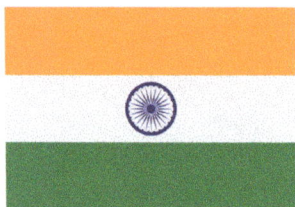

Flags of China and India

Congee and Kichadi

Congee and kichadi are soupy, highly digestible grain dishes. Congee is a typical Chinese breakfast food made with rice, mung beans, and herbs and spices often specifically blended for a person's constitution or ailment. Indian kichadi is similar but usually includes lentils, ghee (clarified butter), and Indian spices.

Congee is also known as zhou (pronounced "jook") by the Mandarin. Another name for congee is shi fan (water rice). Kichadi (aka kitcharee) is used in Ayurvedic medicine to balance the body and is especially recommended for those with deficient or excess "Agni" (digestive fire) and inflamed or irritable digestion. The closest Western counterpart is porridge, which all too commonly contains oats smothered with refined sugar.

Chinese congee shops feature soupy rice congee with a "salad bar" of assorted extras, ranging from steamed vegetables to fish, meat, and eggs cooked by the congee's heat. You may do likewise at home by preparing a hot rice base in a crockpot and serving with a buffet of optional ingredients.

Bob Flaws, in *The Book of Jook*, notes that congee is "...in a form immediately available for digestion and absorption. Rice congee particularly benefits the stomach and intestines. Because it is cooked with so much water, congee helps moisten the fluids of the stomach and intestines that tend to become depleted in old age due to chronic disease. However, it does this without engendering dampness and phlegm." [6]

Congee is nourishing for convalescents, the elderly, and infants. The inclusion of nettles in the following recipe adds a tonifying element and aids the elimination of toxins.

Nettle Congee

1 cup basmati rice*

1 cup sprouted (or soaked) mung beans

6 cups bone broth or nettle water

Spices:

    1 teaspoon fresh grated ginger

    1/2 teaspoon cumin (freshly ground if possible)

    1/2 teaspoon coriander seed

    1/2 teaspoon salt

    pinch asafoetida or black pepper

Vegetables:

    4 cups fresh spring nettles, chopped

    1 carrot, diced (or pumpkin, for variety)

    1-4 cloves garlic, minced

Wash rice well. Place in a saucepan with mung beans, broth or water, and spices. Bring to boil. Reduce heat and simmer covered for 30 minutes. Add vegetables; simmer for 10 more minutes.

*Basmati is generally considered to be the most digestible rice. Many congee devotees alternate organic basmati with brown, black, wild, or red rice for a winter meal.

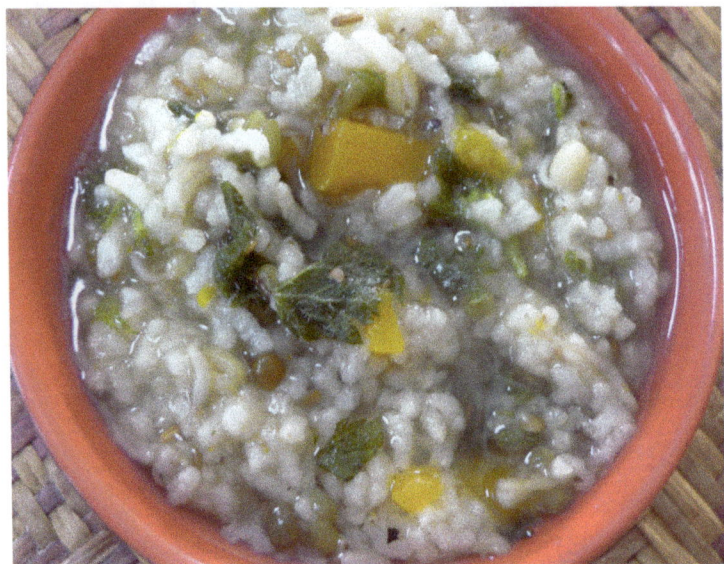

India's Kichadi is quite similar but made with lentils, rice, and ghee (clarified butter). Spices include turmeric, asafoetida, ginger, chili, and vegetables of choice. Ayurvedic practitioners tailor kichadi specifically to a person's constitution and imbalances. Check the internet for a wide variety of kichadi recipes. The addition of nettles provides a profoundly nourishing element.

Nettles & Eggs

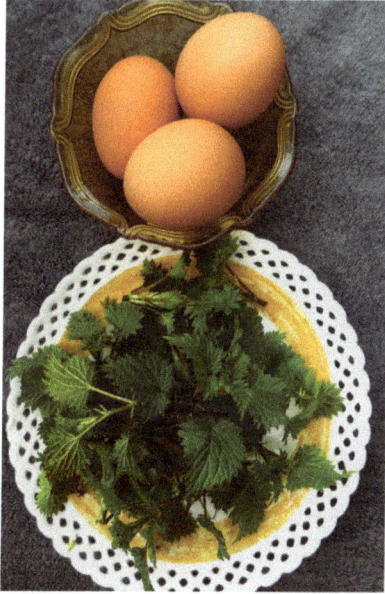

Team nettles with eggs for easy, inexpensive, and nutritious dishes. Add the greens to omelets, soufflés, and quiche. Or layer steamed nettles with poached eggs in an Eggs Benedict type dish.

Substitute nettles for spinach and other greens called for in egg recipes.

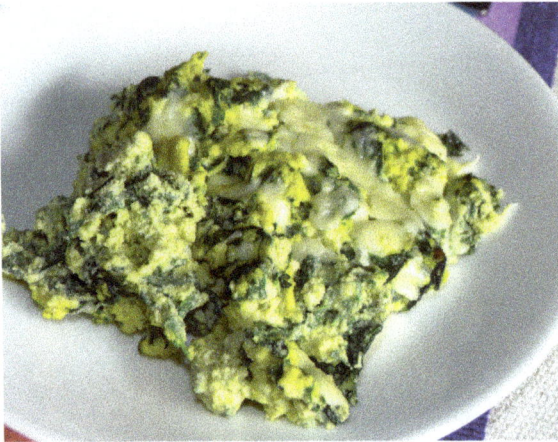

Steamed nettles combined with beaten eggs yield a quick treat equally suited for breakfast, lunch, or dinner. Top with Nesto for extra flavor and nutrients.

Nettle Burgers

Contributed by Elvin Kilcher, HOWL instructor, Homer Alaska

    4 big fistfuls of raw nettles, chopped finely

    2 eggs from your local chickens

    2-3 cloves minced garlic

    1/2 teaspoon each: salt, pepper, onion powder

    dash cayenne pepper

    Extras: oil for cooking, burger buns, condiments of choice

Chop the raw nettles finely. Do not steam the nettles first; just wear gloves while chopping if you don't love the feeling of nettle stings. Mix the eggs, the chopped nettles, and whatever spices you desire in a bowl. The consistency should be gloopy, and you should be able to form 4 loose patties from the mixture.

Heat the oil in a skillet, preferably over an open campfire. When the oil is hot, fry each patty until the eggs are cooked through, and the patty is no longer gloopy.

Serve on a hamburger bun and add whatever condiments you like.

For information about HOWL (Homer Wilderness Leaders) summer camps, visit: www.howlalaska.org

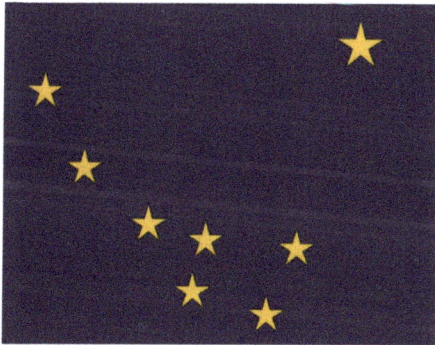

Alaska's flag

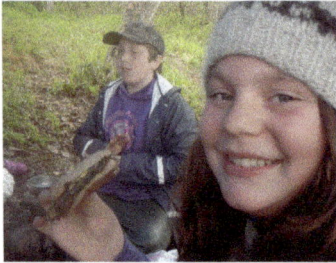

Ella Parks enjoying her nettle burger, with Tim Parks in the background during a Howl outing

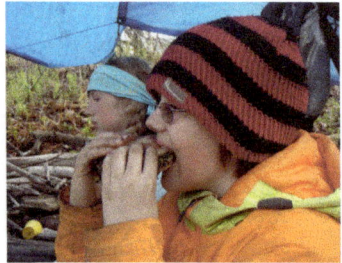

Seamus Schlotz eating his nettle burger with Mia Alexson in the background

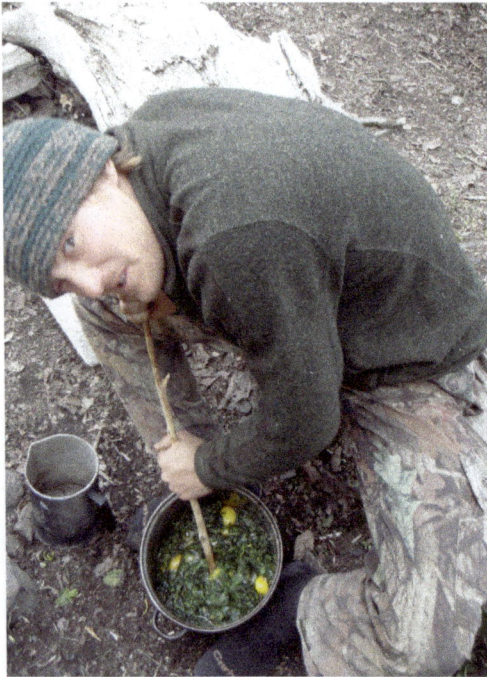

Elvin Kilcher, stirring nettle burgers in the field

Nettles Dips And Spreads

Nettle Cheese Spread

This tasty spread for crackers, vegetable sticks, or sandwiches blends nettles with tangy goat cheese. Serve with Nettle Crackers for a special treat.

1/3 cup goat cheese

1/3 cup in olive oil

2 cloves garlic, minced

2 cups fresh nettles, steamed and drained (save the broth for soups)

Blend all ingredients with a food processor. If using a blender, pre-chop cooked nettles, and add ingredients slowly for thorough mixing.

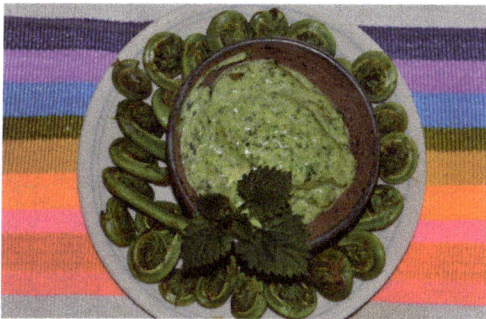

Nettle Dip

Blend steamed nettles with mayonnaise or aioli for dipping sauce for spring fiddleheads or veggie sticks.

Nettle Seeds

Nettle seeds are a nutritious additive to recipes. Add to muffins and other baked goods, or sprinkle with nut butter and bee pollen on toast. Nettle seeds can be wild-harvested or purchased from online suppliers.

Trail Balls

These are a variation of Rosemary Gladstar's famous 'zoom balls.' Nibble as a snack while hiking, working in the garden, or doing strenuous activity.

> 2 cups sesame butter (or other nut butter)
>
> 1/3 cup honey
>
> 2 tablespoons nettle seed
>
> 1/4 cup chopped apricots, dates, raisins, or dry fruit of choice
>
> 1 teaspoon bee pollen (or 1 vial bee pollen -available from a natural food store)
>
> Optional: coconut flakes or carob powder

Blend all ingredients thoroughly. Shape into bite-sized balls. Roll in coconut or carob if desired.

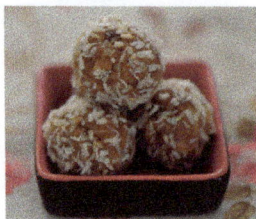

Trail Balls, my must-have for hiking

Saving Nettles For Year-round Use

Drying

When collecting nettles for drying, harvest them in their prime. Collect after the dew has dried but before the day's intense heat. Avoid excess moisture on the nettles.

There are many options available when drying nettles. Tie together in bundles (not too large, so that the inner layers dry thoroughly.) Hang in a warm area with adequate air circulation.

To dry small quantities of nettles, spread on a cookie sheet and place in the oven with a gas pilot light or an electric oven on the lowest setting. I rely on an electric vegetable dehydrator; in prime nettle season, I far exceed an oven's capacity. Dry at temperatures of 41 C (105 F.) for maximum retention of enzymes. Time will vary depending on equipment and method, anywhere from a few hours to overnight.

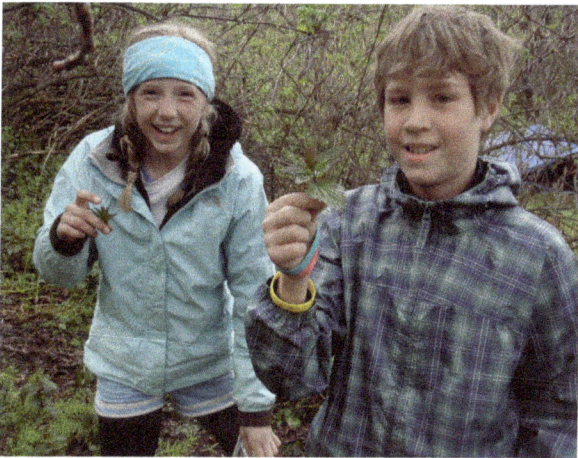

Mia Alexson and Tucker Weston collecting spring nettles

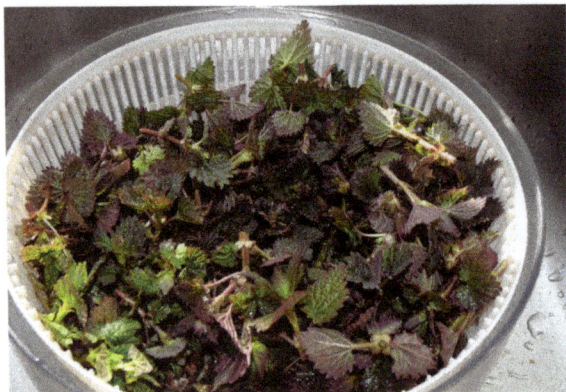

For long-term use, dehydrate young nettles as soon as possible
after picking

I've experimented for years with various drying methods, including the technique used in rainy Southeast Alaska (placing herbs in a sealed pillowcase and spinning in a clothes drier). In bush Alaska, my preferred method for coping with the seasonal nettle bonanza was my wood-fired sauna. I placed clean cotton cloths on the sauna benches and spread them with fresh-cut nettles. Then I lit a fire in the sauna stove, filled the firebox (one time only), and let the fire burn out. The pre-warmed sauna yielded ideal temperatures for drying. With the near-the-floor vents slightly open, an optimum flow of circulating air resulted.

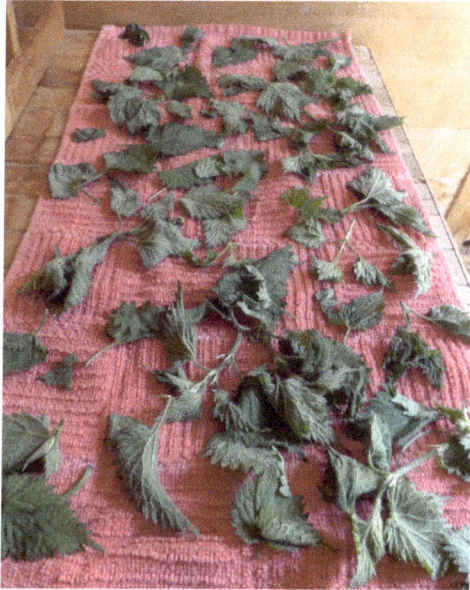

Traditional 'rules' of herb-drying insist on avoidance of direct sunlight. But after sampling the vibrant greenhouse-dried herbs of Andrea and Matthias Reisen of Healing Spirits in Avoca, New York, I've softened my view. "The key to drying nettles in the greenhouse," says Reisen, "is to keep moving them, turning them over. They will dry in less than 24 hours. We lay them out on racks. When dry, they will almost fall off the stems by themselves. A good airflow throughout the greenhouse helps in the drying also."

Henriette Kress lets small nettle bundles swing in the breeze on a sunny day; she reports that they dry quickly, even if pre-boiled, and thus wet.

Preserving Nettles For Culinary Use

In the past, I always preserved nettles for winter use by freezing nettle pesto or pickling nettles. And, of course, I dried nettles for tea. I also added dry nettle leaf (or frozen blanched nettles) to cold-weather soups.

From Henriette Kress, I discovered a new way of enhancing the flavor of dried nettles for culinary use. Dry AFTER pre-boiling (or steaming). "Drying straight," Henriette says, "makes the plant taste more or less like hay."

Try a comparison in the next nettle season, and see which you prefer.

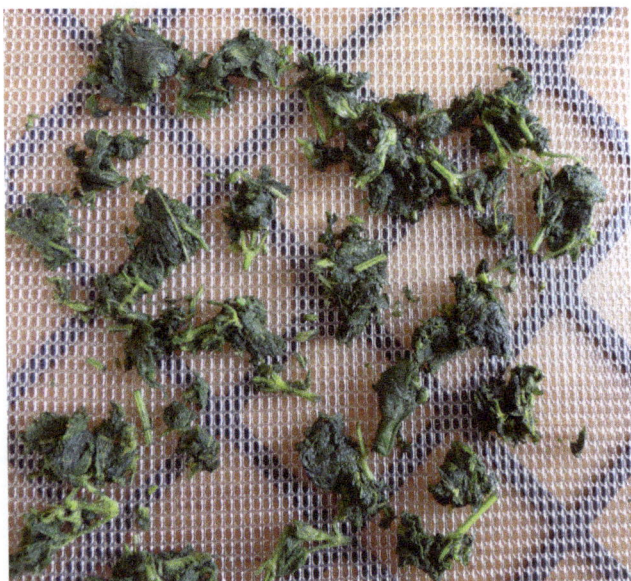

Storing Dried Nettles

Glass jars are ideal storage containers. Label and date your herbs. Store in a dark closet, or wrap sheets of dark paper around the glass to exclude light. Those who lack jars and closet space can store dry herbs in the freezer in double layers of well-sealed and labeled plastic bags. (This method also works exceptionally well for herbs high in volatile oils.) Keep the nettles as whole as possible. If your recipe calls for powdered nettles, grind the herb just before using it to avoid oxidation and deterioration of the nutrients.

Cooking with Dry Nettles

Sprinkle dry nettles in soups. Grind nettles and add the 'flour' to bread and biscuit doughs, crackers, pasta, and seasoning. Use as a nutritional supplement in any dish.

Michael Moore, in *Medicinal Plants of the Pacific West*, wrote: "All over the country, people are taking arcane, obscure food supplements, often with little information to go on and with the side effects and other problems seldom mentioned, and they cost a lot of money. Spirulina and chlorella are algae, dried pond scum that is an excellent food for pollywogs and so high in nucleoproteins (DNR/RNA) that it can cause nitrogen overload, purine buildup, and uric acid excess... Nettle powder is something you can gather yourself in places that you trust... It is green food your body recognizes and can help build blood, tissue, and self-empowerment." [7]

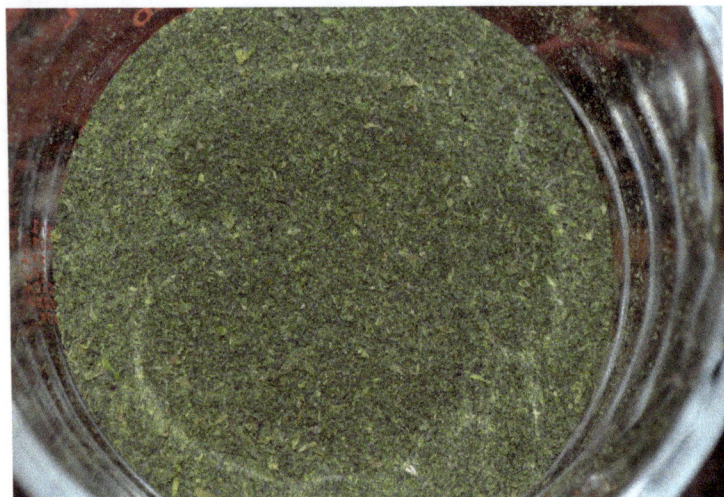

Nettle Beverages

Smoothie Powder

Nettle-powered smoothies are a tasty, fast way to power up your morning. Smoothies are an ideal breakfast, mid-day pickup, or meal-in-a-glass when on the run.

> 5 tablespoons dry nettles, ground and sifted
>
> 5 tablespoons dry, deseeded rose hips, ground and sifted
>
> 1 teaspoon each cardamom and cinnamon powder

Blend ingredients and store in a glass container, labeled. Keep in the freezer to prevent deterioration of herbs.

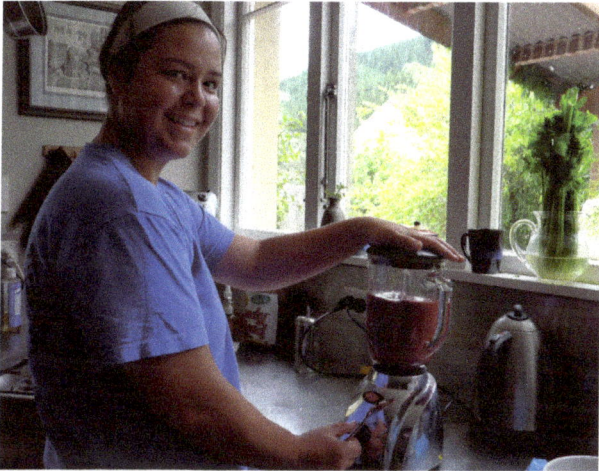

Gayla Pederson of Kodiak, Alaska creating a morning smoothie

Get Up And Go Smoothie

    1 cup milk (nut milk or dairy)

    4 tablespoons probiotic yogurt

    1/2 cup fresh or frozen berries (blueberries, raspberries, strawberries, boysenberries, etc.)

    Optional: 1 banana, fresh or frozen

    1 heaping teaspoon smoothie powder

Place all ingredients in a blender. Blend until smooth and creamy. Thin with milk as desired to adjust for drinkability.

Note: In summer, add extra frozen fruit for an ice cream-like dessert.

Green Zoom

A nourishing green drink inspired by a recipe by Emily Willis, Haines, Alaska.

Some authors use the terms 'smoothies' and 'green drinks' interchangeably. I consider 'smoothies' as milk-based (dairy or nut seed-based), whereas 'green drinks' have a water or juice base.

In a blender, combine:

> 1/2 cup lightly steamed or boiled chopped nettles
>
> 1 cup nettle water (saved from steaming nettles)
>
> 1 handful fresh chickweed tips or cilantro or mint
>
> 1 apple cut in chunks (or 1 cup pineapple)
>
> sweetener of choice (optional)

Cool nettles and nettle water. Puree with remaining ingredients. This recipe is infinitely variable. Options include rhubarb stems, kale, parsley or garden greens, or wild things like lamb's quarter and dandelion leaves.

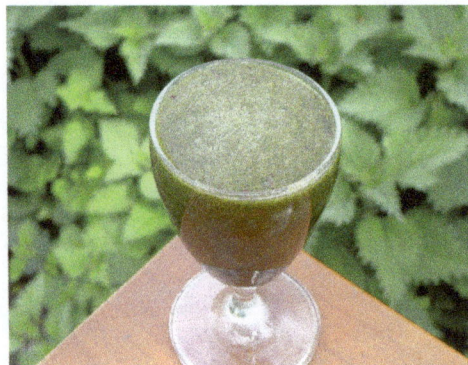

Sweeteners can include fresh pineapple chunks or a bit of honey or a few stevia leaves (or drops of stevia extract), or fresh juice added to the nettle water.

The above 'Zoom' includes nettles with fresh peppermint, chickweed, apples, and a dash of raw honey.

Experiment freely with whatever ingredients you have on hand. My version contained blueberries, parsley, water, and lemon juice blended with the nettles.

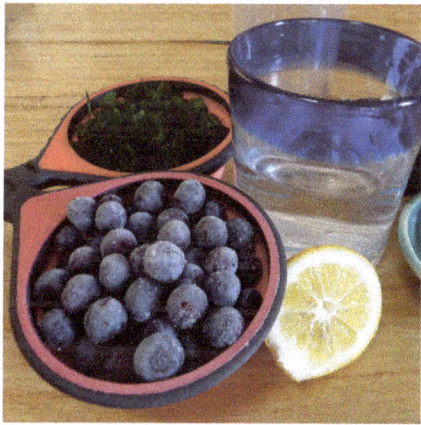

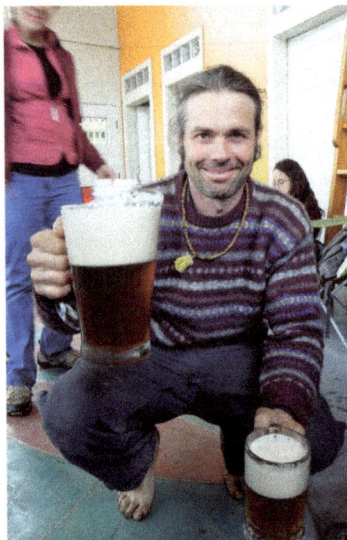

Lasse Holmes sharing his latest
batch of Stinger

Nettle Beer

Cottagers traditionally made nettle beer. Mrs. Grieve, in her classic herbal, wrote that it was given to elders "as a remedy for gouty and rheumatic pains, but apart from this purpose, it forms a pleasant drink." [8] Grieve's statement was unequivocally agreed to by testers of the following beer.

Brewmaster Lasse Holmes assisted me with the creation of the Stinger recipe in 1998. He continued to develop a Nettle Stout that rivals the flavor of Guinness.

"Stinger" is a robust brew, reddish-bronze to dark in hue, with a creamy "mouth-feel" and satisfying aroma. The first taste tests revealed a unique, fresh herbal character. As aging continued, Stinger's flavor ripened and matured.

Tasters were intrigued that nettles were the key ingredient, and all requested additional samples. Creating an even more robust brew may be obtained using two cans of malt extract and eliminating the brown sugar.

Equipment needed:

> Brewing container: a glass 5 or 6-gallon carboy or food grade plastic bucket.
>
> Thermometer: Stick-on strip thermometers (attach directly to brewing container or a standard cooking thermometer
>
> Plastic tubing: Brew shops supply tubing (for siphoning from the carboy to bottles, as well as bottles, bottle cappers, and brewing inspiration.

Note:

1. Before brewing, clean all equipment thoroughly.

2. Use hot soapy water to remove any dirt or residue (or a commercial cleaning solution).

3. Treat with a sanitizing solution, readily available from a brew supply shop. Alternately, for glass equipment, a solution of 2 1/2 Tb bleach per gallon of water can be used.

Ingredients:

> 4 1/2 gallons of filtered cool water
>
> 2 gallons nettle tops

1/2 cup dry yarrow flowers

juice from 2 lemons

2 cups brown sugar (preferably organic)

1 can (3.7 pounds/1.7 kg) unhopped/light malt extract

1/2 package brewing yeast

Place nettles, yarrow, and lemon juice in 2 gallons of water. Bring to boil. Lower heat and simmer for 60 minutes. Strain. Add brown sugar and malt extract and stir until dissolved.

Place 2 gallons of cool water in a sanitized brewing container. Add hot nettle-malt solution. Top with 1/2 gallon cold water (allow room for expansion during fermentation). Add yeast when the temperature is 60 to 74 degrees F. (15 to 23 C.).

Cover container with a lid with a fermentation lock and a towel to protect from light. Store in a warm room (60 to 74 degrees F./15-23 C.) until all bubbling has stopped (5 to 7 days).

Remove scum and sediment by siphoning into the sanitized bucket. Add 1/2 cup brewing sugar mixed with enough hot water to dissolve. Siphon into sanitized bottles. I always use glass for my main batch, but I bottle one beer in a PET plastic bottle.

Note: The plastic bottle allows you to test when your beer is carbonated and able to be transferred from your warm room into your root cellar or refrigerator. When you first fill the plastic bottle, you can squeeze the bottle; when carbonated, the bottle becomes extremely firm. Check daily. (It generally carbonates within seven days when kept in a warm dark place.)

If left too long, the plastic bottle may 'blow its lid.' Glass bottles can also explode, but the plastic is always the first to go and far less challenging than dealing with glass shards.

When the plastic bottle is firm, you can start drinking Stinger or age for up to six months. Store remaining bottles in a root cellar, refrigerator, or cool place.

Arishtas & Asavas

An arishta is an alcoholic Ayurvedic preparation made by decocting an herb and adding sugar. It is traditionally fermented in an earthenware container sealed with clay, smeared with ghee, and covered with cloth layers. The vessel is then buried in the earth to maintain a constant temperature while brewing.

An asava is similar but made with herbs with heat-labile constituents; thus, cold water is used. The sugar in the recipe can be dissolved in boiling water but must be cooled before adding powdered dry herbs.

The ingredients are placed in a vessel and shaken to mix thoroughly before burying.

Arishtas and asanas, and other herbal cordials, are primarily for medicinal (rather than recreational) purposes. The nettle arishta, and nettle balm cordial following, are (when taken in moderate doses by those who tolerate alcohol) a pleasant way of imbibing a tonifying herb.

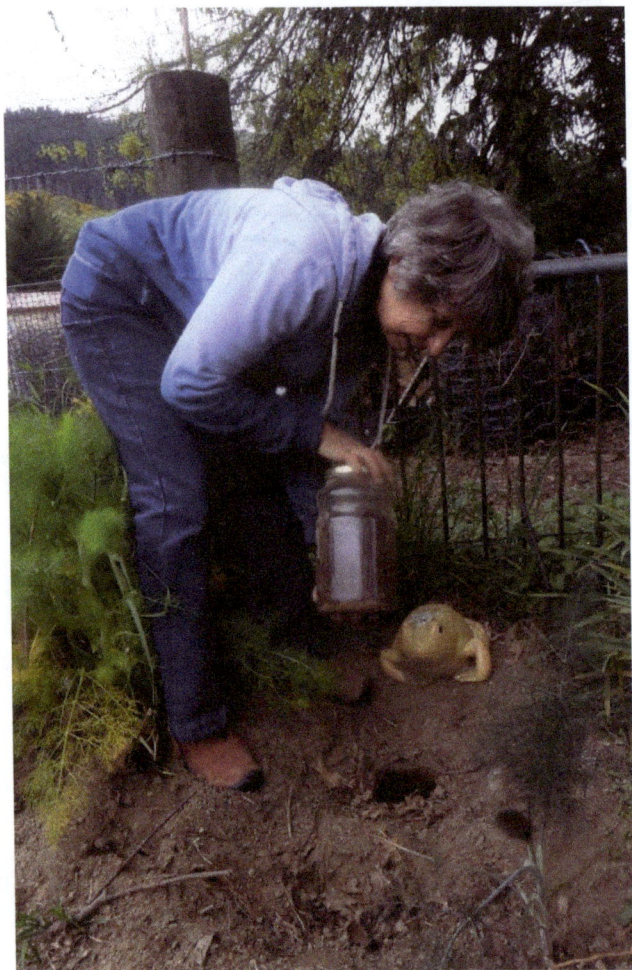

Unburying the arishta

Nettle Arishta

4 cups fresh spring nettles

8 liters (2 gallons) of water

2 cups unrefined organic sugar

Place nettles in cold water; bring to boil. Lower heat and simmer until fluids reduce to 1/2 gallon concentrate. Add sugar and stir until dissolved. Remove from heat. Then place in a sterile glass gallon jar to allow room for expansion while fermenting. Seal the jar well (with clay and ghee if possible) and wrap it in cloth layers. Bury in a quiet place for four weeks. Traditionally, arishtas are unburied at full moon or summer solstice.

When done fermenting, the fluids should be clear and free of any froth. Store in sterile bottles in a cool, dark place. Label. Storage life after opening depends on alcohol content. If 15 percent alcohol, one-year storage life is average. Brewing geeks prefer a hydrometer to measure alcohol content; some brewers trust their 'nose.'

Clinical herbalist Todd Caldecott theorizes that this nettle arishta decreases Vata (see section: Ayurveda and Nettles, for additional details).

My nettle arishta underwent a profound transformation while incubating in the earth. The thin astringent decoction became a sweet/sour syrup with a peach/pear taste.

The dosage for arishtas usually ranges from 3 teaspoons to 3 tablespoons, depending on the herb(s) chosen, the conditions treated, the patient's strength, and the season.

Nettle Balm Cordial

Gratitude to the late Adele Dawson of Vermont, who inspired this recipe and my herbal journey. [9]

2 cups fresh nettles, chopped

1 cup lemon balm, fresh or dried

1 bottle (750 ml.) brandy or vodka

1 tablespoon grated lemon peel

½ cup honey

Combine all ingredients in a glass container. Shake daily for two weeks. Strain, bottle, label, date, and test your patience. I like to give this cordial its debut in the holiday season as a relaxing, healthful, and tasty treat.

Nettle Passion

2 cups nettle leaf tea

1 cup grape juice (white or red)

1 cup mango passion juice

This punch evolved as a special alcohol-free brew for an open house potluck. Blend ingredients in a punch bowl and serve with citrus slices.

For variety, add blueberry or other juices, seltzer water, mint tea, or hibiscus. Experiment freely and enjoy your party.

Nettle Salts and Fermentations

Salt Blends

Emily Willis of Haines, Alaska, reports receiving Lymphatic Salts from a Los Angeles-based herbalist. The blend contained nettle seed, Celtic gray salt, ocotillo leaf, Pacific sea salt, calendula flower, rose petal, violet leaf and flower, cleavers whole plant, dulse, bladderwrack, and kelp. Emily describes it as "a beautiful rose/purple hue and delicious sprinkled on food as you would use regular sea salt."

Sauerkraut and Fermented Nettles

Fermented vegetables are tasty food plus a healing aid for those with leaky gut and digestive issues. Cabbage sauerkraut has long been a favorite of mine, so it's no surprise that I've expanded my kraut to include nettles and other wild greens. Fermented veggies are also great for your immune system.

My attempt to ferment nettles solo was a dismal failure, but ah, combining with cabbage yielded fantastic results. To prepare sauerkraut, you can use a fermenting crock if you wish. I prefer a simple canning jar capped with a fermentation lid (as shown in the following photo). Fermentation lids are readily available on Amazon and other internet sources.

Make sure your equipment is sparkling clean. Boil your container for 10 minutes, or simply place a canning jar in a preheated oven at 320-350 F/ 160-180ºC for 15 minutes.

Ingredients:

   1/4-1/2 nettle tips (freeze to deactivate the sting)

   1 head cabbage - about 3 pounds (1 1/2 kg)

   1-2 tablespoon sea salt

Collect nettle tips and put them on a tray in the freezer. (I do this the night before to encourage complete deactivation of the stinging hairs).

Then prep the rest of the ingredients. Shred or finely chop the cabbage and sprinkle it with sea salt. Give the cabbage-salt combo a thorough massage (with clean hands). Keep pressing (or pounding) the cabbage to encourage it to release its juices.

Remove nettles from the freezer and chop finely or run through a kitchen blender (I used my Ninja). Add to the cabbage and stir in well with a spoon.

Add any extras you desire, such as 1 tablespoon cumin or caraway seed. The inventive batch in the photo includes chopped garlic, grated carrot, chopped spring onion, a dash of harissa, and some magenta-spreen lamb's quarter from my garden for a splash of color. (Chive flowers also add color and flavor).

Press the mixture into a sterile jar (or your crock). The liquid from the pressed vegetables should cover the kraut. If using a canning jar, cap with a fermenting lid. Let sit on the counter for several days, tasting daily. When it tastes 'just right,' refrigerate. Eat a few spoonfuls daily to feed your gut healthful probiotics.

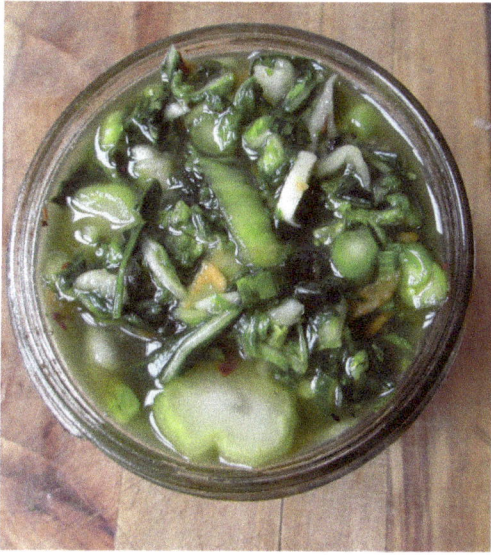

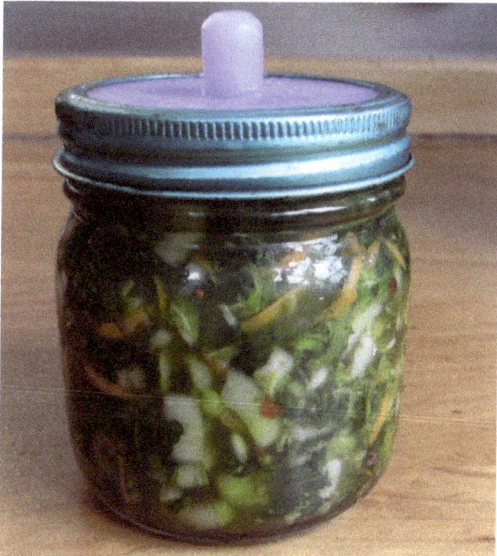

Readers Notes

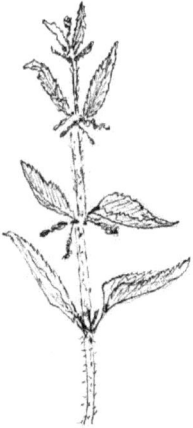

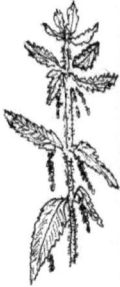

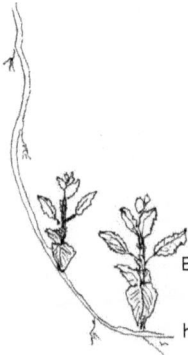

E-mail your new recipes and nettle experiences to:
athomewithjanice@gmail.com
for potential inclusion in the blog:
https://www.athomewithjaniceschofieldeaton.com

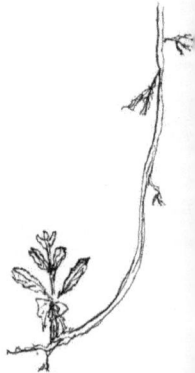

Chapter 3

Cosmetic Uses of Nettles

General Skin Care

Nettles serve as a cleansing agent and wash for the complexion; their astringency makes them especially suitable for those with oily skin. For normal or dry skin, blend nettles with calendula flowers, rose petals, or elderflowers.

Australian author Gail Stern suggests applying a "nettle face" daily for two weeks each spring. To prepare, simmer nettles, whiz into a paste, spread on muslin or cheesecloth, and apply on your face.[10]

Before applying the nettle pack, I like to dampen my face with nettle tea. Place cotton balls over the eyes for protection. Lie back and rest for 15 minutes while the nettle pack nourishes the skin. Rinse well with warm nettle tea combined, if desired, with lemon juice. Finish with a cold water splash to close the pores.

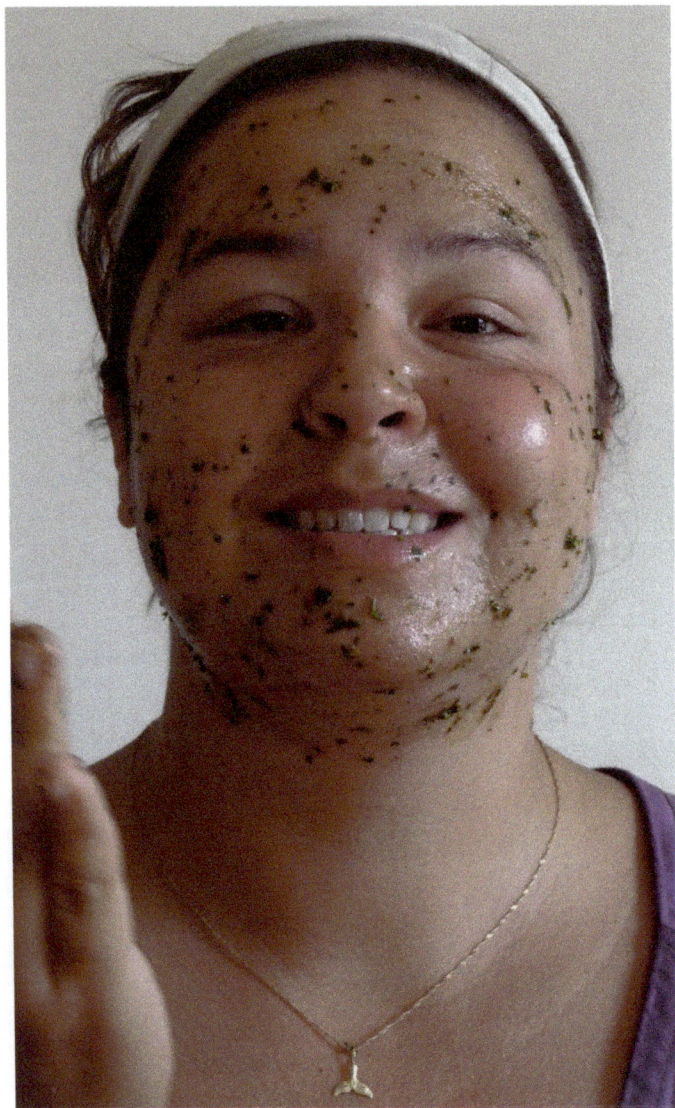

Facial Steams

Nettle facial steams invigorate a dull complexion. Combine with nettles internally for a complete rejuvenation program.

Hair Care

Nettles have a long history of fostering luxurious hair. A Czech study of nettle, chamomile, and thyme verified that the combined extract increased circulation to the scalp and decreased hair oil and dandruff.

German herbalist Maria Treben favors using nettle root tincture, which she rubs ". . . into the scalp daily; even on trips, I take it with me. It is worth the effort, no dandruff, the hair is thick and soft and has a beautiful sheen." [11]

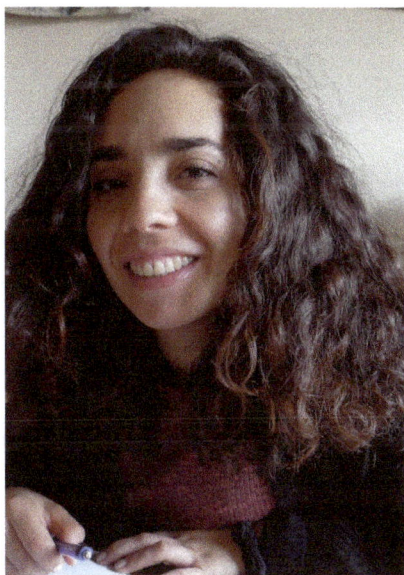

Nettle has a reputation for stimulating the regrowth of hair. Though some individuals obtain remarkable results, nettle is not a panacea for all types of hair loss. Alopecia varies dramatically, from hair shedding in patches or particular areas (from scalp to body hair). Contributing factors range from chemotherapy and hormonal imbalance to genetics, drug use, and nutritional deficiency. If poor nutrition is the culprit, daily nettle ingestion, combined with external application of a nettle wash or lotion, may indeed have a positive effect.

Herbalist Michael Moore recommended nettle seeds as a scalp conditioner and hair-growth stimulant. The seeds contain oils and traces of formic acid. "One teaspoon is soaked in a cup of hot water until lukewarm (approximately 20 minutes); the tea is used as a fine rinse after shampooing." [12]

The following is a luxurious treatment for dry hair.

Nettle Hair Oil

> 1 1/2 cups dry nettle leaf
>
> 1/4 cup nettle seed
>
> 2 cups extra virgin olive oil

Combine ingredients in a glass jar; steep for 3 weeks, then strain and rebottle. Scent with essential oils of your choice, such as rosemary or lavender. Label. Store in a dark cupboard.

Before use:

1. Place 3 tablespoons of Nettle Hair Oil in a teacup.

2. Set the cup in a pan of hot water to warm up the oil.

3. Apply the oil to dry ends.

Far messier, but helpful if your entire hair requires a boost, is to warm 1/4 to 1/3 cup oil and rub thoroughly into hair and scalp. Wrap your head in a towel or swim cap and leave the oil on overnight. In the morning, wash hair well, and rinse thoroughly; shampoo two to three times to remove oil residues.

Nettle Hair Tonic

> 2 ounces nettle leaves,
>
> 2 cups kombucha (or organic vinegar)
>
> 2 cups water (or rosewater)
>
> essential oil of rosemary or lavender

Place nettles, kombucha (or vinegar), and water in a quart (liter) jar and let it sit for 3 weeks, shaking daily. Strain. Scent with a few drops of essential oil. Place in a bottle with a squirt-type lid. Massage thoroughly into hair and scalp after shampooing.

Liquid Soap

My favorite liquid shower and sauna soap (used for both body and hair) is a decoction of nettle, horsetail, and kelp. To prepare, fill a pot with the herbs, cover with water, and simmer gently to a concentrate, reducing the volume to one-third of the original fluids. Blend 1/3 cup concentrate with 2/3 cup liquid Castile shampoo and scent with 12 drops of essential oils of fir needle and rosemary (or other essential oils of choice. Add essential oils sparingly to avoid burning the skin.

Nettle Baths

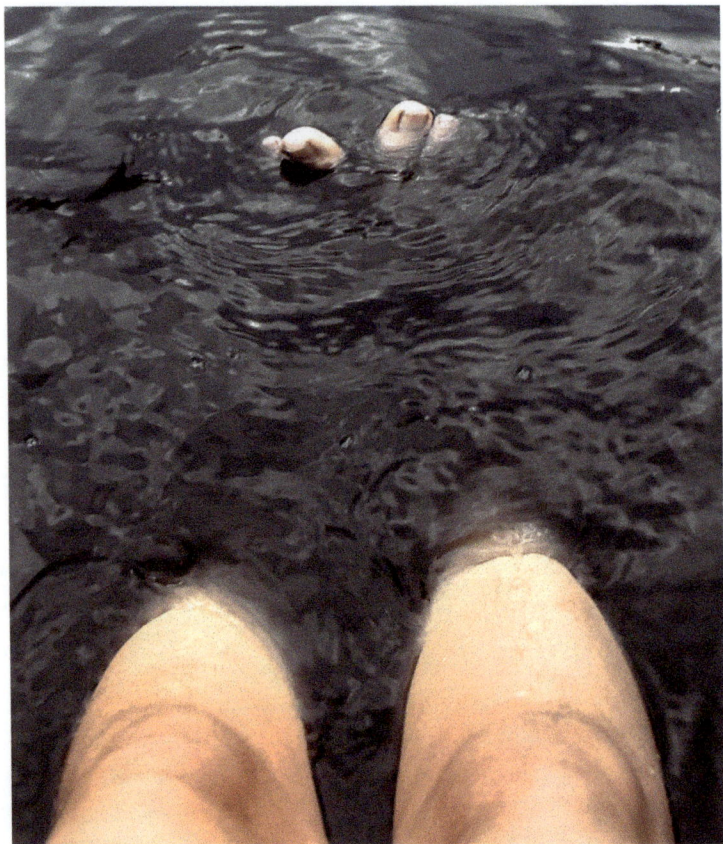

Add nettle tea to your bath for a detoxifying soak. Relieve muscle strain and inflammation. Help ease skin irritation.

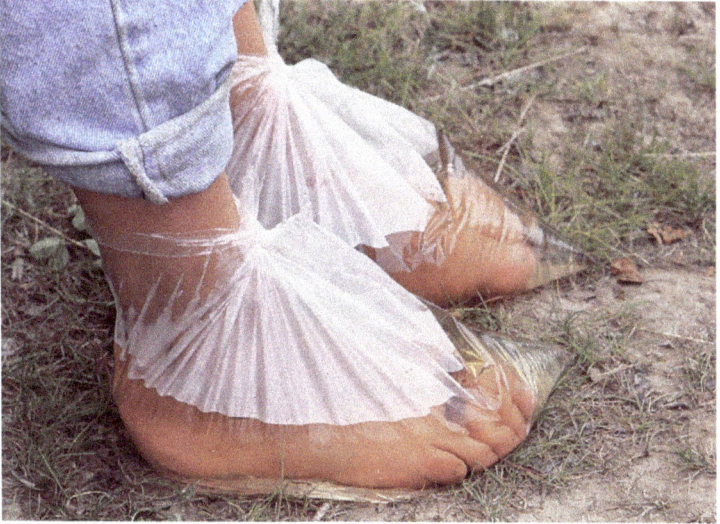

Hikers can indulge in a trail's-end footbath. While sitting around a campfire relaxing, soak sore feet in warm nettle tea. A large zip lock bag makes a handy container (at home, use a basin.). Sip nettle tea while relaxing.

Readers Notes

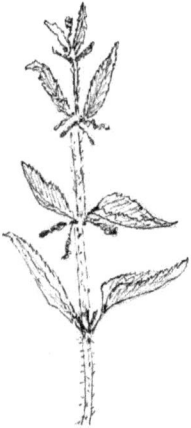

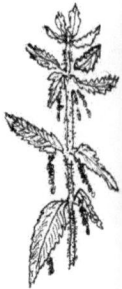

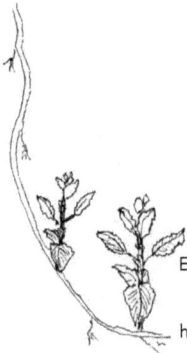

E-mail your new recipes and nettle experiences to:
athomewithjanice@gmail.com
for potential inclusion in the blog:
https://www.athomewithjaniceschofieldeaton.com

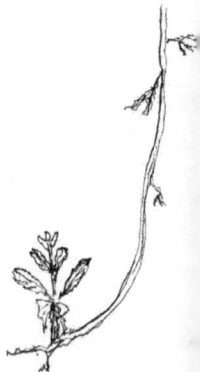

Chapter 4

Modern Medicinal Uses For Nettle

"Everything of the nettle, stems, leaves, flowers, and roots, has medicinal properties."

Maria Treben, Health Through God's Pharmacy

Nettles are so common, safe, and inexpensive to purchase (free if you harvest them yourself) that they are often overlooked. Throughout the ages, humans have tended to value that which is dear or rare. Thus, nettles have garnered far fewer of the research dollars so freely bestowed on more exotic herbs. However, observations made in scientific laboratories concur with those made in the living laboratory of human experience. And nettles endure as a steadfast herbal helper. They are more needed today than ever before to help our bodies cope with the ravages of pollution, stress, and soil depletion.

Nettle Nutrients

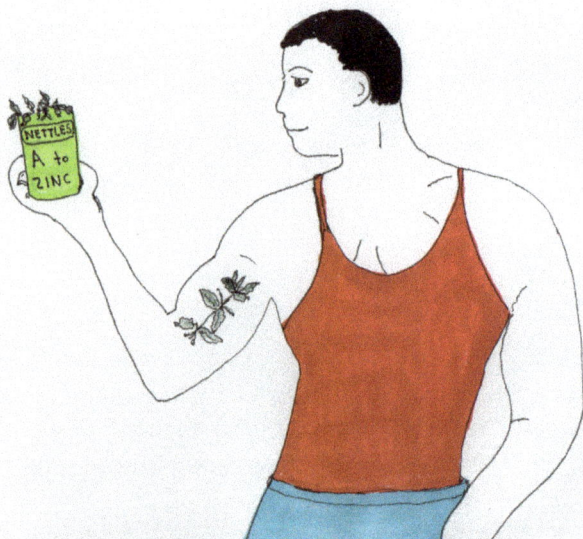

Nettle nutrients far surpass spinach.

Nettles are an extraordinary example of the marvelous complexity of nature and contain a plethora of compounds. The nettle leaf hosts an alphabet of vitamins ranging from beta-carotene (the precursor of vitamin A) to vitamins B1, B2, C, E, and K.

Approximately two cups of steamed nettles equal an orange in vitamin C content (Nettles: 76 mg. per 100 grams).

Of all plants studied by Bulgarian researchers, nettle had the highest nutritional value and most ideal chemical composition. Nettle leaf far surpassed the nutrients of spinach, cabbage, and lettuce. Following nettles in nutrient density were dock and beet leaves. [13]

Nettles are a significant source of essential trace minerals (including bromine, chromium, cobalt, copper, fluorine, manganese, nickel, silicon, and zinc). The *MediHerb Monitor* reports that simmering nettle leaves for 30 minutes yields half as much silicon as a three-hour decoction of horsetail (*Equisetum*). [14] A simple nettle decoction is an easy way to obtain absorbable silica.

Spring nettles contain more ammonium, potassium, and phosphorus; the later summer herb (gather newer growth only) is richer in calcium, magnesium, and sulfur.

Nettle leaves are a significant source of highly assimilable iron. The iron occurs in colloidal form (absorbed in plant tissues), rendering it bioavailable and, in most cases, nontoxic to the body. Natural products consultant Steven Dentali, Ph. D., cautions against harvesting nettles grown on mine tailings or other polluted areas. "High mineral content in some plants that accumulate minerals may have toxic effects." Such contaminated sites should be avoided, of course, for any plant harvesting. (When teaching foraging in the Aleutian Islands, I had to check with residents for appropriate harvesting sites due to past military activity and dumpsites.)

Nettle also contains 16 amino acids. Studies of in vitro tests on digestion document that dried nettles have 11.3 percent digestible proteins. Nettle seeds also contain protein and 26 percent oils rich in essential fatty acids.

Nettles are rich in chlorophyll (the plant pigment responsible for photosynthesis and similar to hemoglobin in structure). During World War II, nettles supplied chlorophyll for medicine.

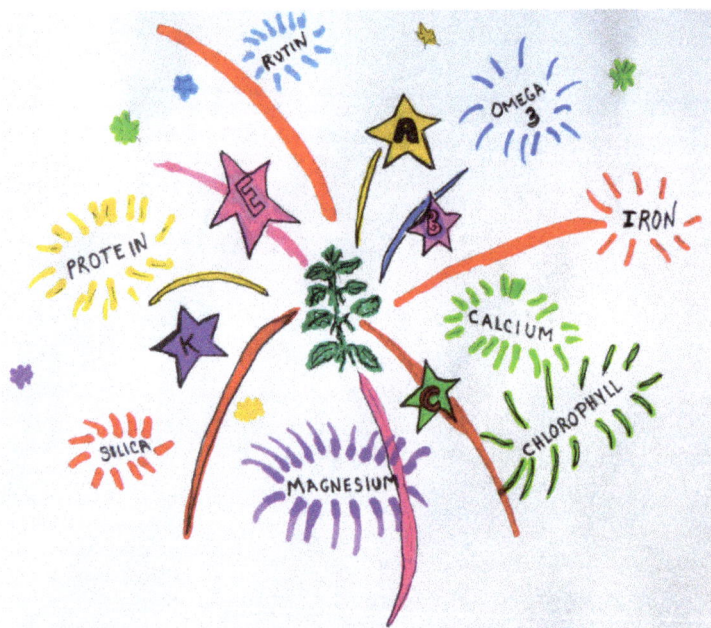

Nettle leaves contain an array of acids and amines, and flavonoids (water-soluble pigments that color plant flowers, fruits, and sometimes their leaves). The nettle's flavonoids are of the quercetin type, which includes rutin. Although this particular flavonoid complex's effects have not been positively documented, antioxidant and anti-inflammatory actions and blood vessel effects are probable.

Tonic, Specific and Low Dose

Robyn Klein of Bozeman, Montana, director of the Sweetgrass School of Herbalism, classifies herbs in three general categories: tonic, specific and low dose. Nettles are both tonic and specific.

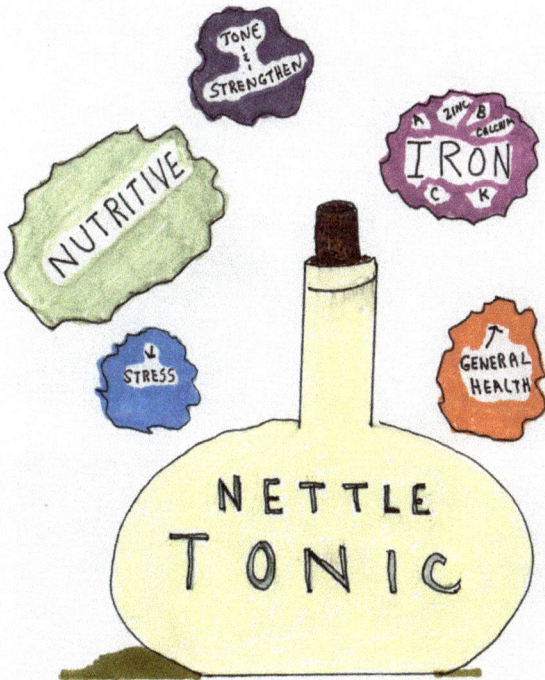

Tonic herbs assist in preventing chronic illness. Like nutritional supplements, their effect is cumulative and safe. Tonic herbs can be consumed for weeks or months at a time. Tonic herbs usually have a propensity for one or more body systems. Alterative herbs also fit in this category as they have an overall beneficial effect on the whole body.

Nettle leaf is an example of a nutritive tonic. It has a particular affinity for the circulatory, respiratory, and urinary systems. The leaf is alterative and enhances vitality and the body's overall functioning.

A 'blood cleanser' is how the ancients described nettle. They noted that drinking nettle tea or ingesting nettles as food for a few weeks benefitted the entire body. Skin problems cleared, allergies eased, and energy increased. They theorized that nettle accomplished these feats by 'cleansing' the blood.

Today, we understand that nettles do not scour dirty blood. If your blood were foul, you would be in intensive care with septicemia. But nettles help eliminate both endogenous (from within) and exogenous (from without) waste metabolites. Leaf infusions have a mild but definite diuretic effect, increasing the excretion of uric acid and nitrogenous wastes.

The German herbal *Drugs and Phytochemicals* by N. Bisset reports that a two-week treatment of nettles increases urine excretion and decreases systolic blood pressure. [15] In addition to supporting the kidneys' eliminative work, nettles enhance the liver and lungs' functioning. These organs are vital in the break-down and elimination of environmental pollutants (including airborne allergens); they are also an essential part of the immune system. Thus, nettles also help enhance immunity.

Specific herbs are, as their name indicates-- specific for an acute illness or condition and usually taken for a brief period (ranging from a few days to a few weeks). Many tonic herbs, including nettles, also have a specific effect and proclivity for a particular

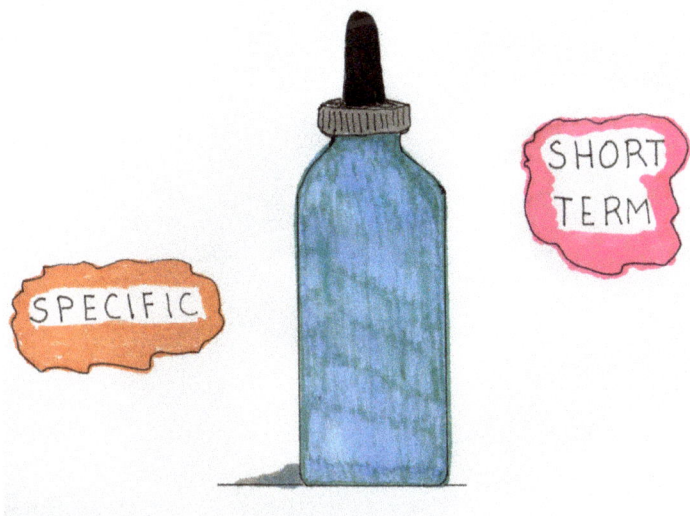

body system or organ. Nettle root is specific for benign prostatic hypertrophy.

Nettle is a safe plant for beginning herbalists as it is a tonic and specific. It does not fall in the category of 'low dose' herbs.'

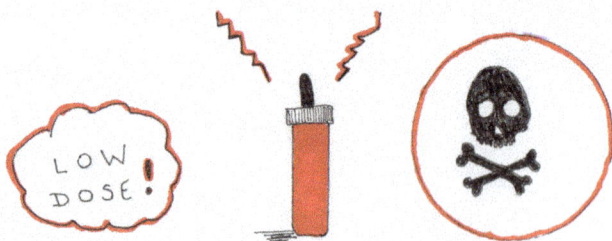

Low dose herbs like wild indigo (*Baptisia tinctoria*) and poke root (*Phytolacca americana*) have potentially dangerous toxicity. Low dose herbs can be used, with care, by knowledgeable practitioners. When used, such potent plants feature as small parts in a formula and rarely if ever given alone.

Depletion and Anemia

Feelings of depletion are common at the end of a long winter. German naturopathic physician Susanne Fischer-Rizzi writes, "I personally swear by a spring course of treatment with stinging nettle to give my body a kick after the winter and chase away fatigue. In fact, the treatment makes me feel like I could uproot a tree!"

Susanne's regime starts with one tablespoon daily of fresh-pressed nettle juice. She increases the dose daily by one table-spoon for two weeks. When she reaches fourteen tablespoons, she switches to decreasing the daily amount by a tablespoon daily until the treatment ends. (The nettle juice may be diluted with water or milk if desired.) She also recommends one to two tablespoons of mature dried nettle seeds " ...as a tonic to

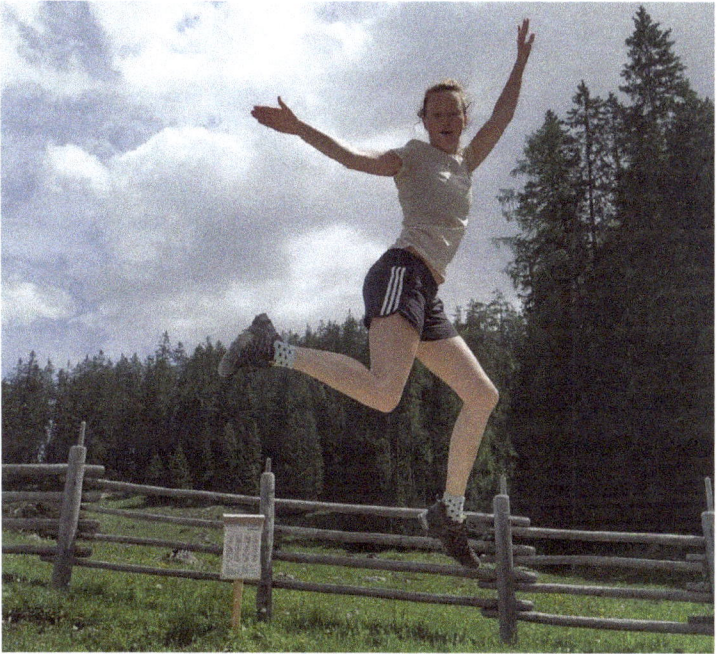

stimulate bodily functions in conditions of exhaustion, in times of stress and during recovery from illness. The seeds are recommended, especially for elderly people." [16]

Weakness, digestive disturbances, or lack of libido can also be due to anemia. Anemia is a symptom complex rather than a disease in itself and is characterized by a reduction in red blood cells, hemoglobin, or blood volume.

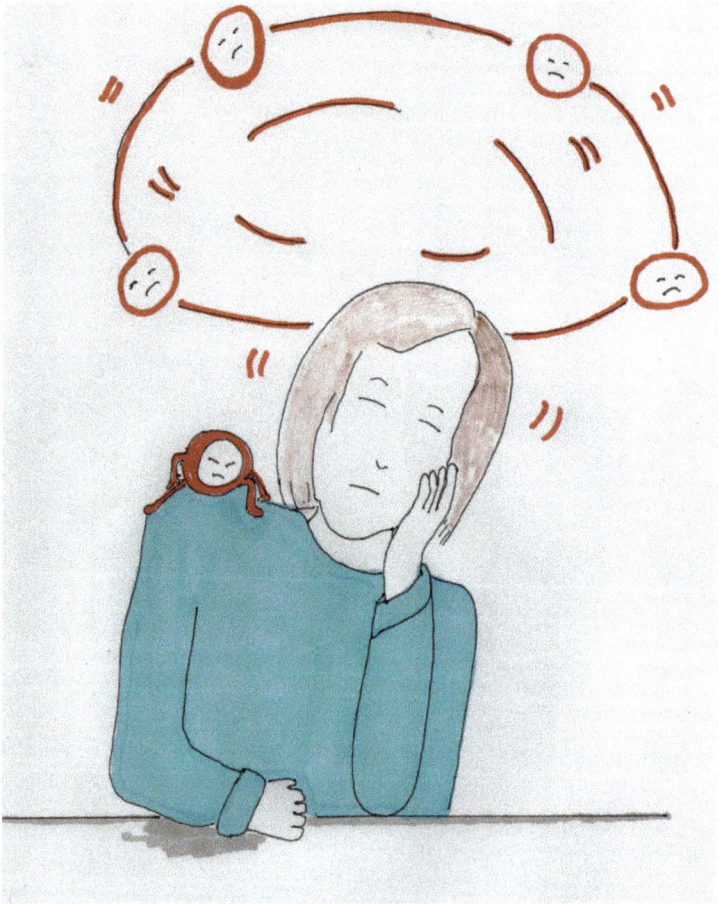

Nettle is specific for anemia due to iron deficiency as the nettle is the richest land plant source of iron. The iron, combined with vitamin C, makes for good absorbability.

United Kingdom herbalist Christopher Hedley prescribes nettle for iron-deficiency anemia most often due to heavy menstrual bleeding, giving birth, and breastfeeding. He recommends four teaspoons per day of nettle Fe extract (an iron-rich 1:1 cold percolated tincture available at herb shops and online). Hedley's wine-based nettle tonic is another helper for anemia.

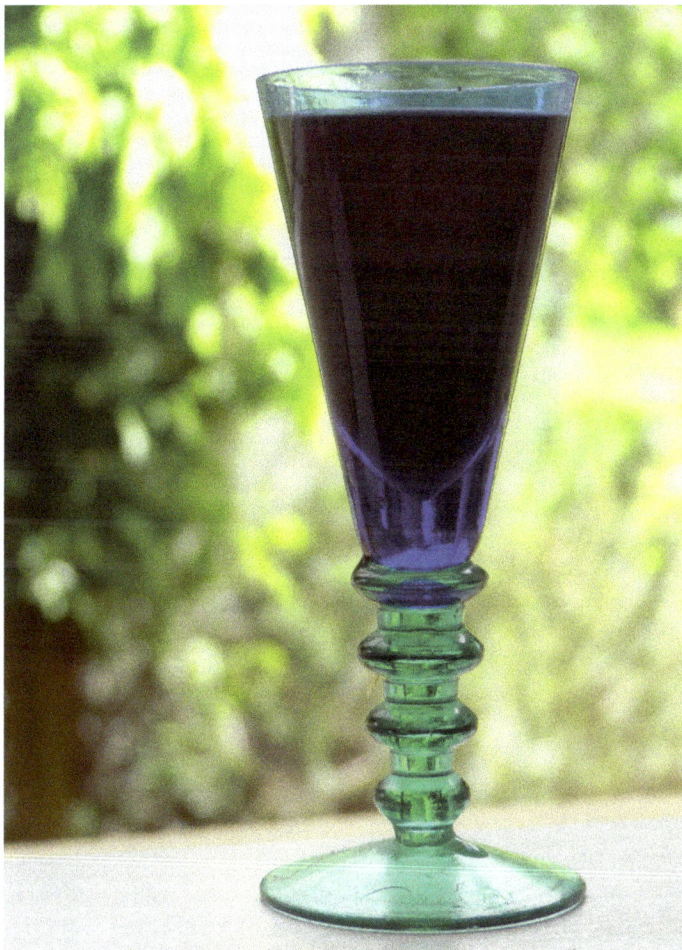

Hedley's Favorite Nettle Tonic

Christopher Hedley's Favorite Nettle Tonic

This tonic brew, says Hedley, is "… nice to make, nice to take, and it works."

Combine equal parts of fresh or dried nettles and dried organic apricots with a handful of unwaxed bitter orange peel. Steep in organic red wine (enough to cover the mixture) for two weeks. Strain and give two teaspoons (10 ml) twice daily.

Hedley uses the peel from bitter oranges (*Citrus aurantium*) in his recipe, as bitters improve digestive function and absorption. Bitter orange, aka Seville or sour orange, is a Southeast Asian native commonly used in marmalade. Chinese medicinal orange peel could be substituted, or if unavailable, use the peel of ordinary organic oranges.

Due to the unavailability of bitter oranges, in my recipe, I used:

   1 cup fresh nettles

   1 cup apricot

   1/2 cup organic orange peel

   enough wine to cover all.

The result was wonderfully fragrant and tasty and a hit at my local herbal group meeting.

Gout and Arthritis

Gout is a type of acute arthritis characterized by joint inflammation. Although it may occur in any location, it usually manifests in the foot (commonly in the toes) or knee.

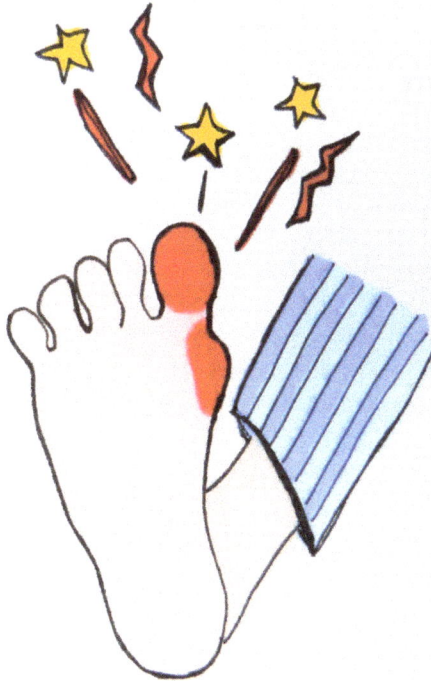

Acute gout attacks often occur at night and progress in intensity throughout the day. The disease is associated with excess uric acid levels in the bloodstream and urate deposits in joint areas. Conventional treatment consists of:

1. Non-steroidal anti-inflammatories such as Colchicine, an anti-inflammatory for acute gout whose side effects may include diarrhea, vomiting, and abdominal pain.

2. Uric acid solvents (such as probenecid and sulfinpyrazone), which may cause skin rashes, nausea, and peptic ulcer aggravation.

3. Xanthine oxidase inhibitors (such as allopurinol), which reduce uric acid formation in chronic gout but may spark fever, skin rash, and hepatotoxicity.

Nettles feature prominently in an herbal approach to treatment. Nettles are a specific herb for gout as they increase the excretion of uric acid and other metabolic wastes. German studies on animals provide supporting evidence of nettle's effects on stimulating the excretion of uric acid, ammonia, and urea.

Australian naturopath Andrew Pengelly uses infusions and fresh plant tinctures of the native nettle (*Urtica incisa*). Pengelly finds this ". . . especially good for arthritis and gout, conditions marked by a build-up of acid metabolites and with histamine-induced symptoms."

The German Commission E monograph validates the use of nettles internally and externally for rheumatic conditions. Nettles have a stimulating action both on metabolic waste excretion as well as absorption of nutrients into tissues. In Germany, nettles are an adjunct treatment for those with rheumatoid arthritis and osteoarthritis.

Besides ingesting nettles for joint inflammation, humans have historically deliberately stung themselves with nettles. Common in the Roman legion participating in military action in damp England, this practice is not as quirky or obsolete as it appears. The soldiers found that the stinging hairs' stimulation eased rheumatic complaints and increased their tolerance to the cold and damp.

A student in my herbal program reported marked improvement in her arthritic hand's mobility after deliberately picking nettle barehanded. Those who wish to receive the benefits of external therapy with nettles without the "itch" can follow the suggestion of Henriette Kress of Helsinki, Finland. Make a sauna 'vihta,' by binding together a bundle of nettles (instead of birch twigs, the usual plant for sauna therapy). Go into the sauna, get a good heat going, and then start hitting yourself with the nettle whip. Henriette says there is no sting; the histamine evaporates before it can cause itching.

The Stinging Hairs of Nettles

The nettle plant bears fine hollow hairs with a swollen, bulblike brittle tip. As the hairs penetrate the skin, the tip breaks, and the hairs release their contents like a hypodermic needle.

Nettle stings have various components, including formic acid, the same compound in the red ants' painful bite.

When injected by a nettle hair (or released from an injured cell), histamine produces the classic red spot and wheal typical of nettle stings. Histamine also increases digestive secretions and dilates capillaries, thus increasing blood flow to the extremities.

Serotonin is a neurotransmitter that plays a significant role as an antidepressant. Serotonin also increases the GI tract's motility and enhances sensory perception. Another nettle sting-related compound is acetylcholine; this neurotransmitter transmits impulses at the junction between nerve cells.

Formic acid, histamine, and serotonin are all water-soluble and all found in nettle infusions and decoctions. When heated, their chemical stabilities are less readily predictable. As for tinctures, histamine and formic acid are soluble in alcohol, serotonin sparingly so.

The physical effects of ingesting neurotransmitters and histamine are not fully known. Evidence shows that when histamine is taken orally (as in eating nettles) and processed through the digestive tract, an antihistamine effect results. (Hence the practice of using nettles for allergies.

As for the impact of the acetylcholine or serotonin present in nettles, much is only currently theory. Howie Brounstein, the owner/operator of Columbines and Wizardry Herbs, reports: "No one really knows how or why this works. It just shows that the gut is a real cross between digestive processes, the immune system, and the central nervous system in ways we are just beginning to understand. The point is, treat the gut in chronic diseases."

Taking serotonin into the stomach is different than increasing serotonin in the nerve synapse in the brain. However, normal gut leakages will cause some serotonin to infuse into the bloodstream.

Is the striking feeling of well-being one experienced when ingesting nettles 'the euphoria of spring'? Is it a brain/body chemical reaction or the result of nettles' nutritional and energetic properties? No definitive answer yet exists. Slowly, we are beginning to decipher the pathways and processes involved. Meanwhile, the plant bears gifts that the mind can't yet fully comprehend.

Skin Problems

Urticaria is a medical term (derived from *Urtica*, the stinging nettle genus) for skin ailments characterized by wheals and itching. Urticaria may be triggered by a wide variety of allergens (including pollens, foods, and drugs) as well as by physical contact with the living nettle plant.

Standard medical treatment for allergy-induced urticaria consists of antihistamine drugs, epinephrine injections, and cortisone. Alternative health practitioners often use homeopathic *Urtica urens* to relieve symptoms, as well as anti-inflammatories such as licorice root (*Glycyrrhiza glabra*).

When the cause of urticaria is physical contact with the nettle plant itself, the tingling and itching generally pass within a few hours. You can hasten the process with applications of jewelweed (*Impatiens noli-tangere*), dock leaves (*Rumex* species), or plantain leaves (*Plantago major*). These herbs often grow in proximity to nettle. Sunny Mavor, the owner of Herbs for Kids in Bozeman, Montana, shared the following nettle story:

"Many years ago, I was on an herb retreat with the California School of Herbal studies. We were backpacking near the Northern California coast when I slipped on a log in a marshy area and fell face-first into a huge patch of nettles. Luckily, they missed my face and eyes, but as I lay face down, I knew that my legs were instantly becoming a hive of welts. I lay in the mud, wondering what to do, realizing that my new-found herbal knowledge was being put to the test. I knew that nettles were placed on this earth for a reason, and for one action, there must be an equal and opposite reaction. As I pushed my way up to a sitting position, I grasped some *Equisetum* (horsetail) for balance. It popped apart at the joints, and inside was a gooey, slippery liquid that must have at one time been water. This goo, growing right next to the nettles, was the perfect cure. I've intentionally used it since, and it has always worked."

While leading a natural history tour with ten Australians, I had the opportunity to test the horsetail treatment. An elderly naturalist, intent on birdwatching, tangled with a nettle patch. I crushed horsetail stems and smeared the inner fluids on the irritated area. The stinging swiftly subsided.

Rubbing nettles (between gloved hands) also yields an inflammation-relieving juice. Convincing someone to apply nettle juice to nettle-irritated skin, however, can be quite a challenge. I've personally done this countless times with excellent results.

Acne, Eczema, and Psoriasis

Eczema is an inflammatory skin condition and, like anemia, describes a pattern of symptoms rather than a disease itself. Eczema is often associated with exposure to specific substances like chemicals, external allergens or genetic factors.

Nettle is an excellent support herb for any acute or chronic skin ailment. In France, nettle leaf infusions are a treatment for mild to moderate acne. Take freely as a daily tea (1 to 3 cups) or juice (1 to 3 tablespoons). Insect bites, scratches, and skin sores all benefit from nettle juice, tea, or ointment.

Fresh-pressed juice is laden with chlorophyll and other nutrients and is a soothing preparation externally for skin ailments. Add 10 percent grain alcohol or 25 percent brandy to preserve the nettle juice. An easy alcohol-free method is to freeze nettle juice in ice cube trays and thaw one as desired.

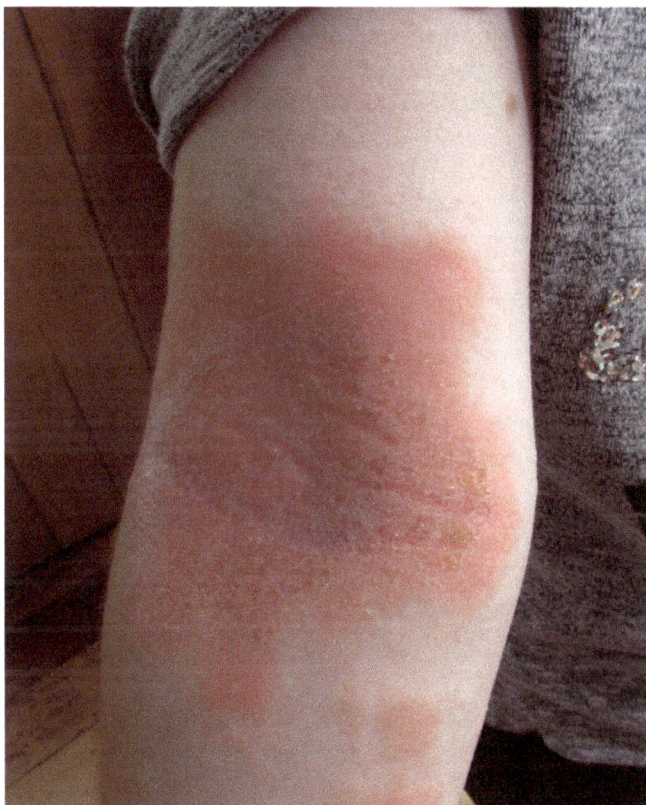

Yet another method, favored by herbalist Christopher Hedley, is to strain fresh-pressed nettle juice well, heat gently to body temperature, skim well, and store in an airtight sterilized bottle. Hedley also recommends "...eating very 'pure' for ten days (mostly vegetables and some fruit, no animal products, sugar or alcohol) and drinking large amounts of herbal teas (especially nettles and cleavers)."

Human blood must maintain a slightly alkaline pH. Most body waste products are acidic. Herbalist Michael Moore wrote: "Nettle tea helps to add electrolytes and alkali to assist the buffering system when under stress, and nettle specifically helps increase the transport and excretion of blood-nitrogen waste products. This makes it very useful in arthritis, eczema, and psoriasis-particularly when the problem is aggravated by anxieties, freakouts, or really bad food (and combinations thereof)." [17]

Poison Ivy

Frank Cipriani, a survival skills teacher in the Pine Barrens of New Jersey, discovered the therapeutic benefits of nettles for poison ivy through his mishaps with the latter and his fondness for eating nettle greens. "I used to get poison ivy seven to eight times a year," says Frank, "I tried all the remedies."

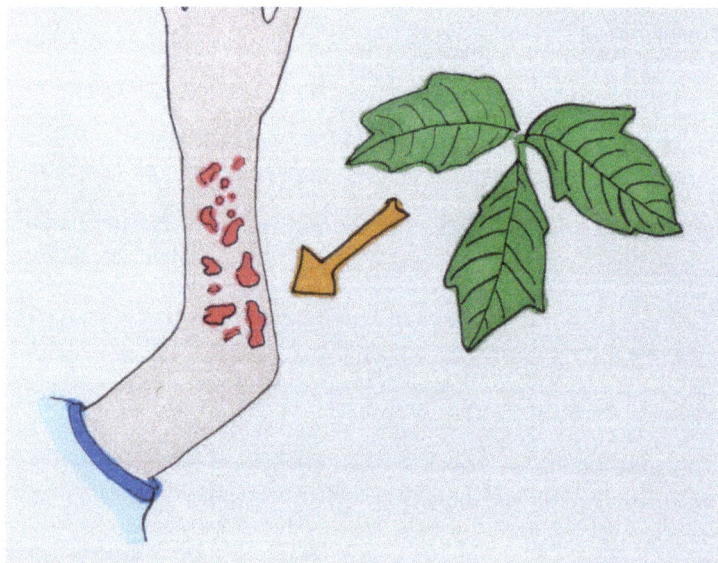

Cipriani found that eating plain boiled nettles, and drinking three cups of the cooking fluids daily as tea, cleared even the most stubborn poison ivy case within three days. He recommends rest and avoidance of sugar and stimulants during the treatment. He theorizes that nettles would be of use in any allergic-type response where the body's reaction may be worse than the toxin itself.

Lupus

Lupus is a chronic skin disease more common in women than men, characterized by a scaly rash that may be limited to the face or body. The disease may progress to systemic lupus erythematosus, an autoimmune condition involving inflammation of the joints, kidneys, and skin. Allopathic treatment generally involves corticosteroids, salicylates, or antimalarial drugs. In all cases of lupus, avoid sun exposure.

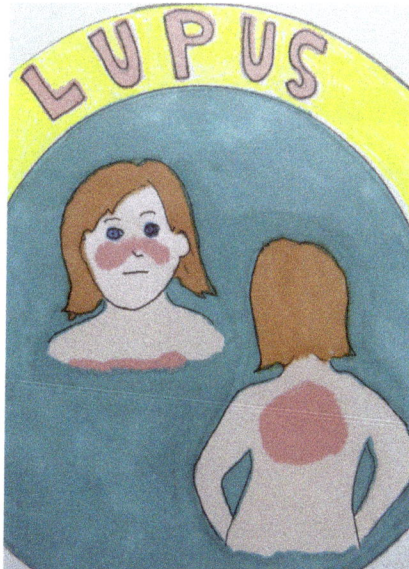

Though nettle is not a cure for lupus, it may play a role in easing the symptoms. Studies reported in the *European Journal of Immunology* indicated that *Urtica dioica* agglutinin inhibited the development of systemic lupus erythematosus-like pathology. [18] (Erythema is Greek for redness and refers to the rashlike symptoms characteristic of lupus. In many cases, this includes a characteristic butterfly rash on the facial cheeks.) Unfortunately, this study was limited to mice, and its effects on humans with lupus require further research.

Bleeding

Nettle is astringent (tightening to tissues), making it a fine choice for inhibiting the bleeding of hemorrhoids. A cotton-tipped applicator may be immersed in a strong nettle decoction and applied to the anal canal. Make a poultice for wounds or mild burns with the pounded steamed herb. The tannins in nettles combine with the proteins in the flesh, creating a protective layer resistant to infection and irritation.

Nosebleeds, spitting up blood from the lungs or upper intestinal tract, bleeding ulcers, and stomach hemorrhage are among the conditions listed by Fisher and Painter as responding to treatment with nettles. [19] Sprinkle nettle powder on shaving cuts to aid coagulation.

Herbalist David Winston uses nettle root clinically for mild menorrhagia cases (excessive bleeding during menstrual cycles) and mucus discharges, bladder prolapse, and blood in the urine. Winston points out that the cause of bleeding (such as stones tearing a ureter, a tumor, or a trauma) must also be addressed.

Urinary Tract Infections

Consider using nettles for chronic urinary and kidney/bladder diseases. The German Commission E monograph approves nettle infusions for lower urinary tract inflammation and renal gravel treatment. In New Zealand, the rhizome and herb are used in the treatment of chronic cystitis.

A 'kidney food' is how clinical herbalist David Winston describes nettle seed. Low back pain, male infertility, and dizziness are regarded as deficient kidney conditions in traditional Chinese Medicine. Winston uses nettle seed for these conditions, as well as degenerative kidney ailments. He combines mullein seed and nettle seed ". . . for people with severely diminished kidney function, and glomerulonephritis (inflammation of the filters in the kidneys). He reports decreased inflammation in five of six patients. The one that did not respond was a woman with approximately twenty percent kidney function left and severe liver disease, both induced by chronic alcohol consumption.

Respiratory Health

Nettles have a long history of use to prevent and treat hay fever and allergies and adjunct therapy in asthmatic care. Nettle has antispasmodic and expectorant qualities. A double-blind clinical study using freeze-dried nettle extract for allergic rhinitis treatment demonstrated a mildly positive response compared to the placebo.

In the experience of herbalist Laura Krieger, daily use of nettles in diverse forms-- food, tea, capsule, and tincture "...has reduced my seasonal allergies amazingly, especially when taken in conjunction with echinacea. It seems to keep my head clear of sinus congestion."

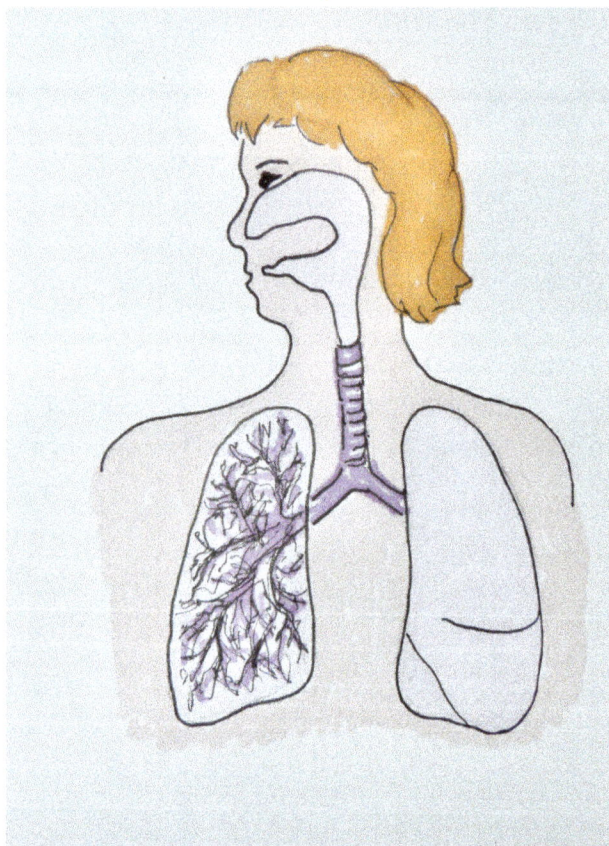

Richo Cech of Horizon Herbs utilizes "...a liquid extract of nettles (composed of a mixture of extracts of the mature seed, dormant root, and immature fresh aerial portions) for treating allergies. It contains histamine and tends to mediate hypersensitivity. Therefore, the burning and itchy eyes and frequent sneezing associated with an allergic reaction to natural allergens such as pollen or hay dust or unnatural allergens such as cigarette smoke and pollution may often be remedied by the daily use of this extract.

As with many natural cures, consistent use of small quantities of the extract may prevent allergic episodes quite reliably, while taking 'megadoses' during an attack may provide no relief whatsoever. You have to trust that it will work, remember to take it, and give it time."

Michael Moore of the Southwest School of Botanical Medicine considered nettle a 'synergistic decongestant.' Nettle increases the effect of herbs such as Ma Huang (*Ephedra sinesis*) and reduces the quantity of ephedrine herbs or preparations needed. (lessening the occurrence of ephedrine-related hypertensive reactions). Moore found that nettle combined well with "allergy-head-cold-coughy-wheezy-red-eye type herbs," including eyebright, goldenseal, and yerba mansa. Nettle seeds, added the late Michael Moore, "...are an excellent lung astringent, particularly useful after bronchitis and such, to return tone and capillary strength to the bronchial mucosa." [20]

While revisiting Alaska in spring after a long absence, I began experiencing respiratory and nasal congestion and fatigue. It finally dawned on me that the 'allergy symptoms' coincided with my low nettle intake. Ordinarily, in springtime, I consume nettles daily. This season I'd been on the road and away from nettles. After arriving in Homer and gathering and eating abundant nettle greens and taking nettle tincture, I quickly experienced respiratory relief.

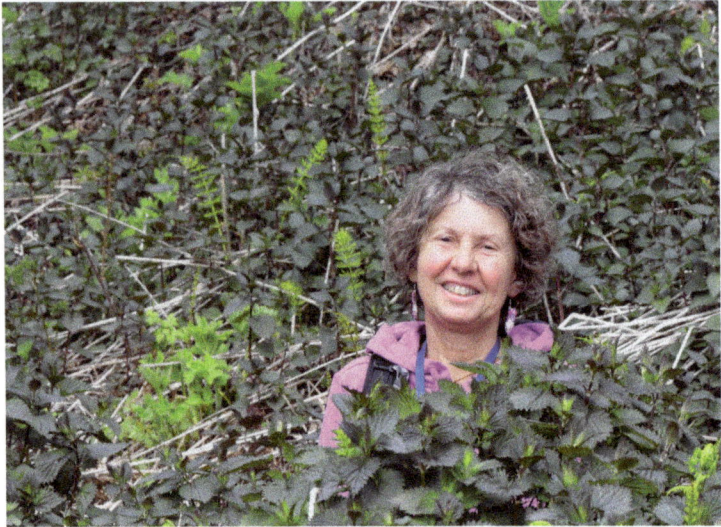

Premenstrual Syndrome (PMS)

Premenstrual syndrome is a complex condition. It involves inter-
actions between the female organs, hormones, liver, digestion,
and the brain's neurotransmitters. Excess estrogen and deficient
progesterone are typical of the most widespread form of PMS.

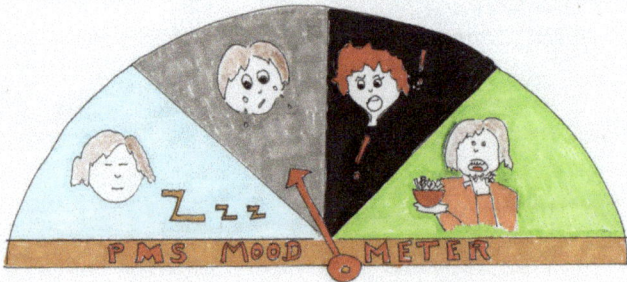

Symptoms commonly include emotional highs and lows, breast tenderness, a 'buddha belly,' and irritability.

There are many factors at play as to why PMS is on the rise, affecting half of the menstruating women (some 15 percent severely). One aspect (associated with the high rate of prostatitis in men) is the addition of estrogen to livestock feed. Since the liver plays a vital role in converting and excreting hormones, facilitating proper liver function is essential. A holistic approach includes switching to organic grass-fed and free-range meats and wild and organic greens, fresh fruits, and regular exercise.

Paul Bergner, the editor of Medical Herbalism, reports that stinging nettle (*Urtica dioica*) is a "...useful herb for PMS, not specific for the liver or the estrogen balance but great for general detoxification.

Nettles are nutritive, astringent, and diuretic (reducing bloating and breast tenderness.) Bergner recommends half burdock root, half nettle leaf tea as an excellent beverage for use during PMS. Nettle, especially when consumed as food, says Bergner, "...is an excellent source of magnesium, an essential cofactor for the enzyme system in the body that transforms active estrogen into its excretable form. Magnesium is so vital that sometimes supplementation alone will significantly improve PMS. An ounce of nettle leaf contains 286 mg of magnesium, more than half the daily requirement."

Pregnancy

Nettle, harvested when young, is a nourishing drink for pregnant women. Combine with raspberry leaf to tonify the reproductive organs. Avoid when the plant is flowering as it can be irritating to kidneys and a possible uterine stimulant. It is also best to avoid the concentrated extract during pregnancy.

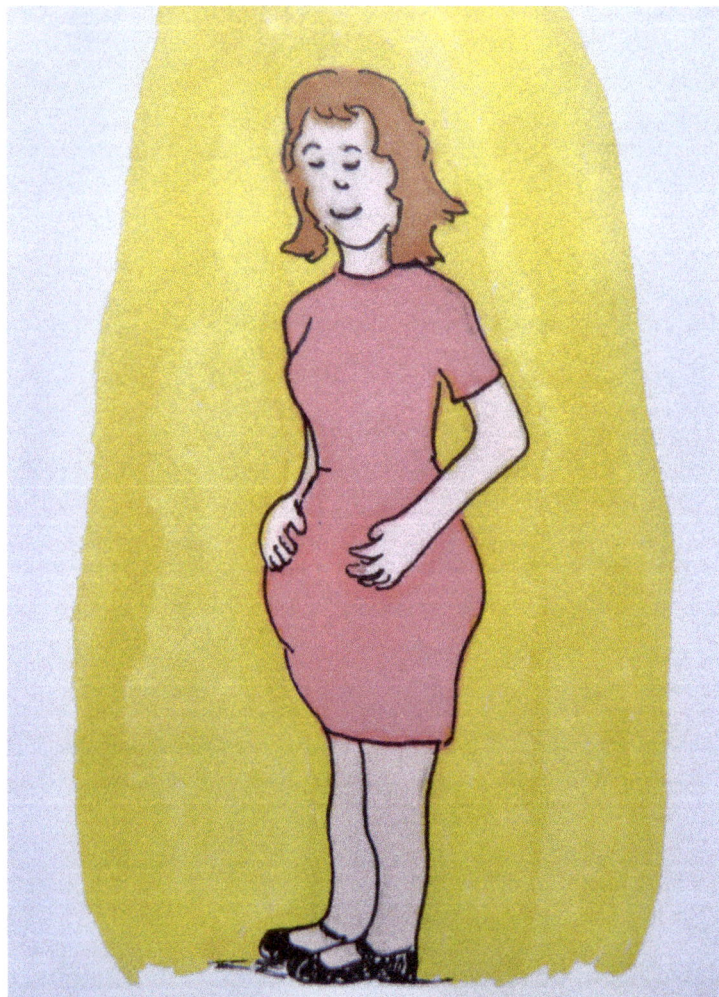

Women report that drinking nettle tea throughout pregnancy and lactation yields enriched breast milk. Include nettles in nourishing food dishes throughout pregnancy. The abundant nutrients aid the growing baby. Many reports show that the mother's food during pregnancy will affect the growing child's food cravings—what better food to crave than nettles.

Herbalist Rosemary Gladstar states that nettle "... is virtually a pregnancy tonic by itself." Drinking nettle infusion before and throughout pregnancy:

Nourishes and strengthens the kidneys.

Increases fertility.

Nourishes the mother and the fetus.

Diminishes leg cramps and childbirth pain.

Preventing hemorrhage after birth.

Reduces hemorrhoids.

Increases the richness and amount of mother's milk.

Prostate Health

The prostate is a walnut-sized structure that is part muscle, part gland, and found only in males. The urethra (urinary canal) arises from the bladder, passes through the prostate, and extends through the penis to the tip. Within the prostate, the urethra forks; this branch has its origins in the seminal vesicle, a structure that lies adjacent to the bladder and produces a fluid that mixes with sperm. Before ejaculation, the prostate adds milky fluids to this viscous soup of semen.

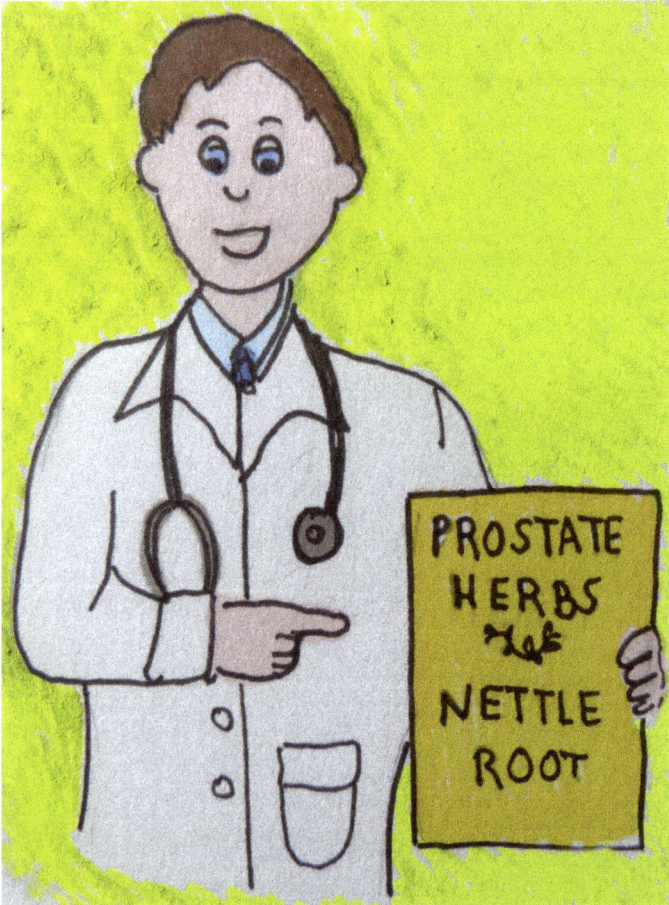

Benign prostatic hypertrophy, commonly called BPH, is an enlargement (often progressive) of the prostate gland. This enlargement can affect the ability of the tubes lying within it to transport and excrete urine and semen. BPH is a common condition in males over fifty years of age. It is often noticed when the quantity of urine diminishes and the frequency of urination increases. The urine stream may be harder to start or longer to pass. Pain may occur with ejaculation. If BPH progresses, the bladder may not empty completely, and residual urine may stagnate, leading to urinary tract or kidney infections.

Finasteride (Proscar) is a drug often used in the treatment of BPH. It inhibits the enzyme 5-alpha-reductase, thus inhibiting dihydrotestosterone conversion, which is associated with triggering BPH. The drug is considered marginally to moderately effective and has side effects, including impotence, in some users. In advanced BPH cases, surgery to restructure the section of the prostate gland impinging on urine flow may be essential to avoid uremia and kidney damage. Annually, 350,000 men undergo this surgery. Its risks include bladder infections, bladder perforation, urinary incontinence, and impotence.

In Poland, in 1993, a clinical study was conducted with 134 males, 53 to 84 years of age, with benign prostatic hyperplasia. Half the participants received two capsules daily, containing 300 mg. *Urtica dioica* (European nettle) root extract combined with 25 mg. *Pygeum africanum* bark extract. The other half received a half-dosage of the same herbal preparation.

After 28 days of treatment, both groups noted significant improvement. Symptoms of Nocturia (frequent urination during the night), urine flow restriction, and residual urine (due to the bladder not emptying properly) all decreased. There were no dropouts from the clinical study due to side effects. As the trial continued, both groups continued to note decreased urinary frequency at night. Interestingly, the half-dose group had an additional markedly significant improvement in residual urine after 56 days. [21] Higher dose does not necessarily equate to better results.

Fisher and Painter note that "the rhizome seems to block the binding of androgens to sex hormone-binding globulin. Treatment was most effective after three months usage and before the enlargement becomes fibromatous." [22]

Herbalist David Winston prepares nettle root as a 1:5 tincture and prefers the recently dried root over the fresh. In a personal communication, he wrote: "It works well with *Serenoa, Salvia apiana*, and *Collinsonia* for the spectrum of prostatic disorders. I believe it potentiates the *Serenoa*; the two work better than either one by itself." *Serenoa* (saw palmetto) is a scrub palm common in the southern United States. The medicinal fruits are theorized to block 5-alpha-reductase or affect estrogen binding in the prostate.

In clinical trials comparing saw palmetto's effects and that of Proscar, Serenoa has demonstrated significant success. [23] Winston adds that "aromatic (fresh leaf, flower, and root tincture) are specific for venous congestion and stagnation with irritation. White sage (*Salvia apiana*) helps to shrink a swollen prostate, reducing discomfort and dysuria."

There are many factors at play in disease, and BPH is no exception. Prostatic enlargement is associated with testosterone accumulation (which converts to dihydrotestosterone and increases cell growth and enlargement). James Green, herbalist for Simpler's Botanical Company and author of *The Male Herbal*, theorizes that "testosterone is a hormone that helps keep healthy aggression intact. When a male retires from his professional work, he often loses an arena for his normal constructive, active aggression, so he needs to keep his lifestyle active to keep from being too retired. This may help him avoid accumulating excessive testosterone in the prostate gland." [24]

Maintaining an active exercise program and eliminating hydrogenated fats in the diet benefits both heart and prostate health. Nutritionally, supplementation with zinc has also demonstrated its usefulness in reducing prostate enlargement. [25]

In Conclusion

The programs described above involve nourishing self-care. They are not a magic bullet. But herbs sometimes act magically, especially when combined with other positive health practices.

If a health problem arises, by all means, get a proper medical diagnosis. Understand your ailment's mechanisms. Weigh both the risks and benefits of conventional and alternative treatments. Illness also offers an opportunity for soul-searching. Examine your lifestyle and create step-by-step changes to restore balance. The nettle is but one strong thread in the weaving of a healthier life.

This edition of Nettles was finalized during the Covid pandemic. Nettle, though not a cure for Covid by any means, can help boost the immune system. In clinical trials, nettles have demonstrated anti-viral properties. One study by Kumaki and others, done on mice, showed the effect of a lectin in nettles inhibiting replication of the SARS-CoV virus.

From a nutritional standpoint alone, nettles are a powerful aid to enhance immunity or recover from illness. From a financial perspective, foraging nettles yourself for food and health helps ease the economic strain of lockdowns and lost jobs. Foraging wild plants becomes vitally important when people need to 'do more with less.' Sharing this wild superfood is my gift to help everyone thrive healthwise and economically.

Readers Notes

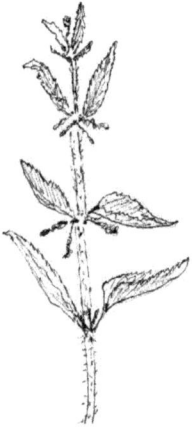

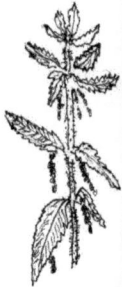

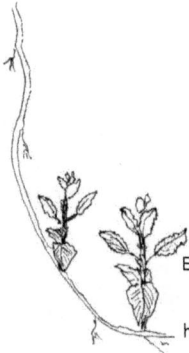

E-mail your new recipes and nettle experiences to:
athomewithjanice@gmail.com
for potential inclusion in the blog:
https://www.athomewithjaniceschofieldeaton.com

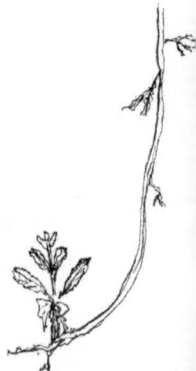

Chapter 5

Nettle Health Preparations

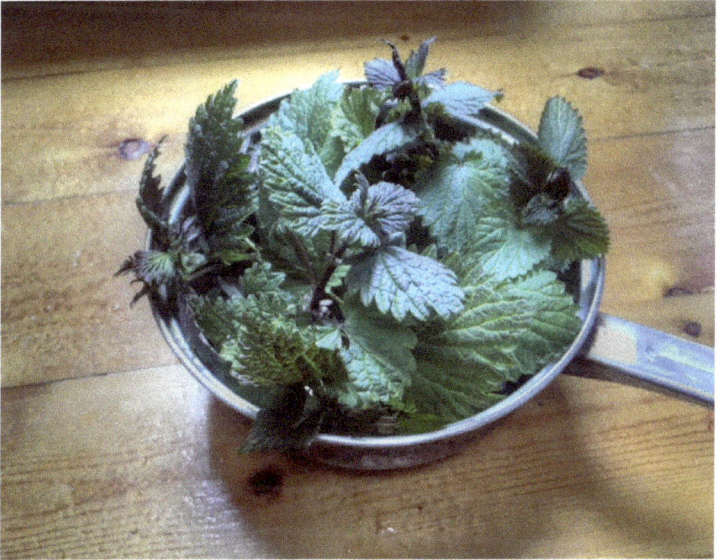

"Yao shi tong yuan"
Medicine and food have the same source.

Japanese proverb

Infusions and decoctions are water-based herbal preparations. With an infusion, constituents are extracted by steeping the herb in hot or cold water. Infusions are effective for easily water-soluble components like leaves, flowers, fleshy fruits, and soft aromatic roots (like valerian).

To prepare a decoction, place the herb of choice in cold water. Bring to a boil, and simmer gently on low heat (usually 15 to 20 minutes). Decoctions are the standard method for denser materials like most roots, seeds, and bark.

Anyone who has ever steeped a tea bag in water has technically prepared an herbal infusion. However, the common name 'tea' generally refers to pleasant-tasting mild herbal beverages drunk for pleasure and recreation. 'Herbal infusions' refer to brews containing herbs deliberately chosen for medicinal intent. Infusions are brewed longer (typically 10 to 20 minutes rather than the 3 to 5 for a tea). The quantity of herb used is also often greater than for a 'tea.'

Hot Infusions

Hot water infusions have a long and revered history. They are the most popular method for leafy herbs and are quick and easy to prepare. Boil water, remove from the heat and pour over the herb of choice in a standard teapot. Or you can infuse the herbs in a glass jar with a lid (to prevent oils from escaping). I prefer the latter method for herbs with delicate, volatile oils.

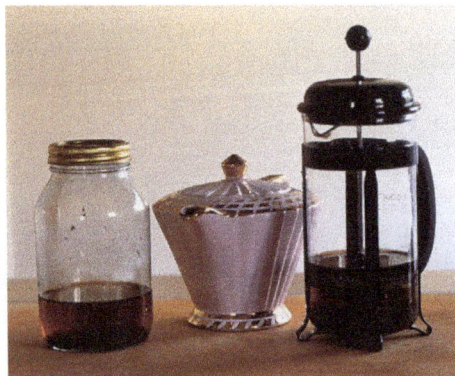

Hot water nettle infusions are very pleasant to drink and a bit earthy in flavor. Some prefer nettle spiked with a touch of mint.

Making sun tea is another way to prepare a hot nettle infusion. Add 1 tablespoon nettle leaf per cup of cool water in a glass jar and place on a hot sunny windowsill for 6 to 8 hours. The sun heats the water and extracts the herbal constituents. Results taste more similar to a 'hot' infusion than a cold.

Hot Nettle Tea

Place 1 tablespoon nettle leaf (fresh or dried) in a teapot or glass jar with a lid. Cover with 1 cup of boiled water. Steep 15 minutes. Strain and serve.

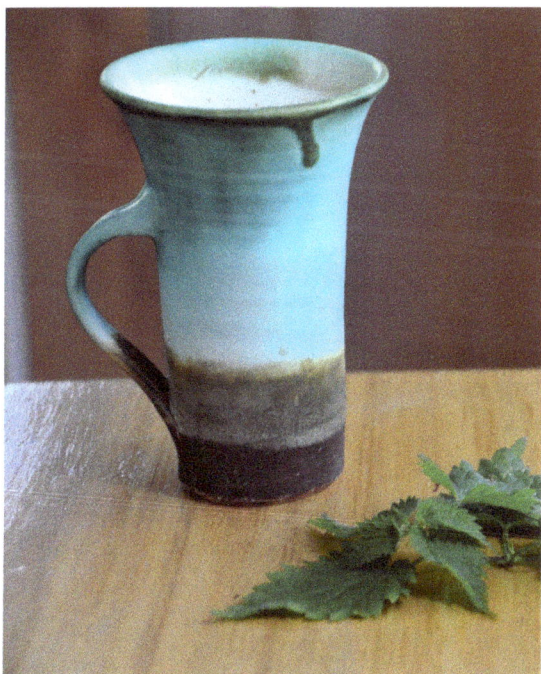

Cold Infusions

Infusions prepared with cold water, in my opinion, are vastly underused and under-appreciated. Cold effectively extracts delicate, volatile oils (such as in peppermint) and mucilage (the slippery, soothing, slimy substance found in okra, chickweed, fireweed stems, and marshmallow root). Cold water infusions (sometimes referred to as 'macerations') do best with at least 8 hours of steeping.

Note: Cold water infusions should be avoided by those with impaired immunity (as in HIV) due to possible bacteria on the herbs, which would be destroyed by heat.

Cold water infusions of nettle are light, refreshing, and convenient. While camping in Tasmania, my backpack contained home-sealed nettle teabags. Each evening I placed one teabag (approximately 1 tablespoon nettle leaf) in a small thermos, topped by 1 cup of cool water. I began each day with my cool nettle brew. Throughout my travels, I felt incredibly energized and vibrant.

Moon teas, prepared by steeping herbs in cool water in the light of a full moon, are another type of cold water infusion. They carry a unique quality that I find incredibly energizing.

Bountiful Blend is pleasant as an anytime 'pick-me-up' suitable even for elders, children, and pregnant women. If purchasing dried herbs in bulk, buy 1/2 ounce of rose petals and 1 ounce of the remaining herbs.

Bountiful Blend

> 2 cups nettles (*Urtica* species)
>
> 2 cups oat tops or oat straw (*Avena sativa*)
>
> 4 cups red clover blossoms (*Trifolium pratense*)
>
> 2 cups raspberry leaf (*Rubus idaeus*)
>
> 2 cups lemon balm leaf (*Melissa officinalis*)
>
> 1 1/2 cups spearmint (*Mentha spicata*)
>
> 1/2 cup rose petals (*Rosa species*)

Blend herbs and store them in a glass container (a gallon jar works well). Label. Store in a cool place out of direct sunlight. To prepare, place 3 heaping tablespoons in a wide-mouth jar or teapot. Cover with 3 cups of boiled water. Steep 15 minutes. Strain. Flavor with honey or lemon if desired. Place in a thermos and sip throughout the day. This tea is also excellent served cool; mix with juice if desired.

Nettle Decoctions in Milk

Australian clinical herbalist Andrew Pengelly suggests decocting nettles in milk since warm milk is high in tryptophan, which is the usual dietary precursor to serotonin. Use 1 tablespoon dry nettle leaf (or 2 tablespoons fresh) and simmer gently in 2 cups milk for 15 to 20 minutes.

Shelf Life of Infusions and Decoctions

When taking infusions therapeutically, I find it easiest to brew a quart or more at a time. Place your day's brew in a thermos and refrigerate any excess. Rewarm as desired or drink at room temperature. (Avoid ice-cold beverages as they inhibit the digestive process.) The shelf life for refrigerated teas is generally 48 to 72 hours.

Make sure to filter your infusion or decoction well to extend shelf life. Discard immediately if a souring taste or murky physical appear. These are indicators of the tea going bad.

Nettle Root Decoction

Place 2 tablespoons chopped nettle root in a saucepan. Cover with 2 cups of cool water. Bring to a boil. Lower heat and simmer covered for 20 minutes. Strain and serve.

Syrups

The word syrup is from the medieval Latin *siropus*, to drink. You create a syrup by blending herbal infusions, decoctions, juices, or fluid concentrates with a sweetening/thickening agent. Syrups are soothing and excellent preparation for inflamed or irritated mucous membranes of the throat, bowels, intestines, or lungs. Syrups are typically tasty and readily accepted by children, elders, and those with picky appetites.

The shelf life of syrup is generally 6 to 8 weeks. Following is a recipe for Nettle Nutritive Syrup. For a pregnant woman or

a young girl entering puberty, substitute raspberry leaf for the alfalfa.

Nettle Nutritive Syrup

1/2 cup dried nettle leaf (*Urtica* species)

1/2 cups dried alfalfa leaf (*Medicago sativa*)

1/2 cup astragalus root (*Astragalus membranaceous*)

1/2 cup red clover blossoms (*Trifolium pratense*)

1/4 cup dried rose hips (*Rosa species*)

Place herbs in a saucepan with 24 ounces of water. Bring to boil. Lower heat and simmer covered until the water level has reduced to approximately half. Strain the herbs through muslin or cotton cloth (a clean flour-sack dish towel works well). Discard the pressed herbs. Measure the fluids. To each cup of herbal decoction, add 1/3 cup honey or 1/4 cup vegetable glycerine. Store refrigerated. Take 1 tablespoon before each meal.

Another Nettle syrup option:

Blend nettle tincture with 3 parts simple syrup for a quick, easy syrup. To prepare simple syrup, stir 1/4 pound honey in 1/2 cup water until well blended. Heat gently until well mixed, being careful not to burn.

Then add 1-ounce nettle tincture per 3 ounces of simple syrup. (Nettle tincture may be purchased at a health food store or made easily at home; recipe following).

Tinctures

A tincture (often referred to as an extract) is an herbal preparation using ethyl alcohol (brandy, vodka, grain alcohol) or
vegetable glycerin or vinegar as a solvent. Vegetable glycerin is
a sweet, syrupy product obtained by distillation of a fixed oil,
such as almond. Obtain glycerin from natural food suppliers
or by mail order. Most herbalists prefer vegetable glycerin to
glycerin of animal origin (a by-product of the slaughterhouse
industry).

Alcohol Tinctures

Alcohol (combined with water) dissolves the broadest range
of plant constituents. With nettles, 80 proof alcohol (i.e., 40
percent alcohol, 60 percent water) works effectively. Brandy and
vodka are typically 80 proof (divide proof by 2 to determine
alcohol content; the remainder is water.)

Note: Resinous herbs, such as myrrh (*Commiphora molmol*) and
cottonwood buds (*Populus balsamifera*), need a strong solvent like
grain alcohol (150-195 proof, 75-95 percent alcohol) to dissolve
the resins. Nettle's constituents extract easily, thus dilute with
water to 80 proof range if using grain alcohol.

When preparing tinctures, many herbalists rely on the moon
cycles rather than a standard calendar. For example, I often start
my remedy at the new moon and strain and bottle at the full
moon. You may even wish to leave the tincture in the moonlight
for the last few days. (During the day, bring back into the house
and keep out of direct sunlight.) In my experience, teas infused
in full moonlight are extra potent and energizing.

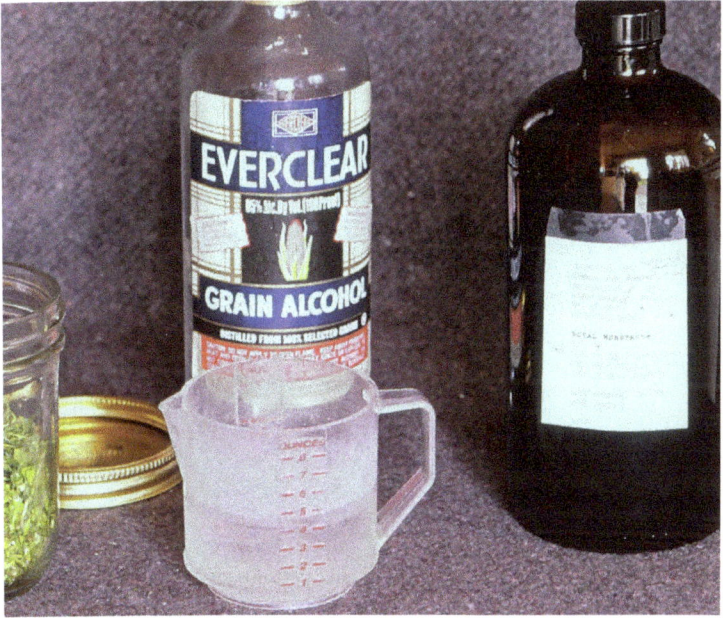

One of my students reported success setting her tinctures in a hot water bath and having them ready for use within 48 hours. Though I prefer the slower, more conventional method, this might be an attractive option if sudden illness strikes.

Nettle Leaf Tincture: Simpler's Method

This method of tincture-making works especially with freshly dried nettle leaf.

> 1 cup dry nettle leaf
>
> 1 1/4 cup brandy or vodka

Place nettle leaf in a jar. Cover with alcohol and press firmly to fully immerse the herbs. Label and date. (I store tinctures-in-progress near my toothbrush as a reminder to shake twice daily.)

After two to three weeks, strain, discarding herbs back to nature. Rebottle fluids, preferably into a clean, dark-colored glass jar. Label. The standard dose is one teaspoon two to three times daily.

Note: If using fresh herbs in your tincture, choose higher strength alcohol, such as 100 proof vodka, to compensate for the water content in the plant.

Ratio Method of Tincture-Making

The "Simpler's Method" of covering the herb with alcohol was standard for centuries. Those who prepare herbal tinctures for the market, or clients, generally prefer a more 'exact' method of weighing the herb and menstruum (solvent) for a more consistent result. For herbal tinctures prepared with dry herb, this is usually a 1:5 ratio, that is, 1-ounce herb per 5 ounces solvent. For fresh herbs, the ratio is typically 1:2 (due to the fresh herb's water content).

Nettle Root Tincture (Ratio Method)

1 ounce recently dried nettle root, chopped

5 ounces 80 to 100 proof vodka or brandy

Steep two to three weeks, shaking daily. Strain through a muslin cloth, pressing well. Compost herbs. Rebottle fluids in a dark glass jar. Label.

The standard dose for a 150-pound adult: 1 teaspoon three times a day. As a petite elder 45 pounds lighter, I reduce my personal dosage to ½ teaspoon three times a day. Consult with an herbalist if uncertain of your ideal dose.

Glycerin Tinctures

Glycerin tinctures work particularly well with mints, fennel, licorice root, chamomile, and other aromatic herbs. Use 60 percent glycerin and 40 percent water. Nettle also works well as a glycerite and ideal for individuals who prefer to avoid alcohol.

Nettle Leaf Glycerite

2 ounces freshly dried nettle leaf, crushed or powdered

7 ounces vegetable glycerin

5 ounces distilled, reverse osmosis or spring water

Place nettle leaf in a wide-mouth quart (liter) jar. In a bowl, blend glycerin and water thoroughly; pour over nettles and mix well with a wooden spoon.* Shake twice daily for two to three weeks. Strain through muslin or cheesecloth. Compost herbs and rebottle fluids.

Standard adult dose for nettle glycerite: 1/2 to 1 teaspoon three times per day.

*When preparing a glycerine tincture, make sure to immerse the herbs fully in the solvent to prevent mold. Depending on how 'fluffy 'the particular herb is, you may need to add extra solvent. Use the same ratio of 60 percent glycerin and 40 percent water.

Vinegar tinctures

Vinegar is a common solvent, especially for tonic herbs. Vinegar tinctures are adaptable. Take by drops or add to salad dressings and marinades.

Spring Tonic Tincture

> 1/2 cup chopped fresh nettle
>
> 1/2 cup chopped fresh dandelion leaf
>
> 4-6 cloves minced garlic
>
> 6-8 chive blossoms, chopped
>
> 1 1/2 cups organic rice or apple cider vinegar

Place herbs in a wide mouth glass jar. Cover with warmed vinegar and seal with a lid. Shake twice daily for two weeks. Strain and label.

Use as a salad dressing. (If desired, blend with extra-virgin olive oil, lemon juice, seasonings of choice) or take 1 teaspoon daily.

Fire Cider is an immune-boosting vinegar-based tonic of spicy and nutritive herbs. Countless variations exist on the internet. My own version is ever-changing, but one basic (besides the typical horseradish-ginger-chili) is spring nettles. The tonic in the following photo was made with kombucha vinegar.

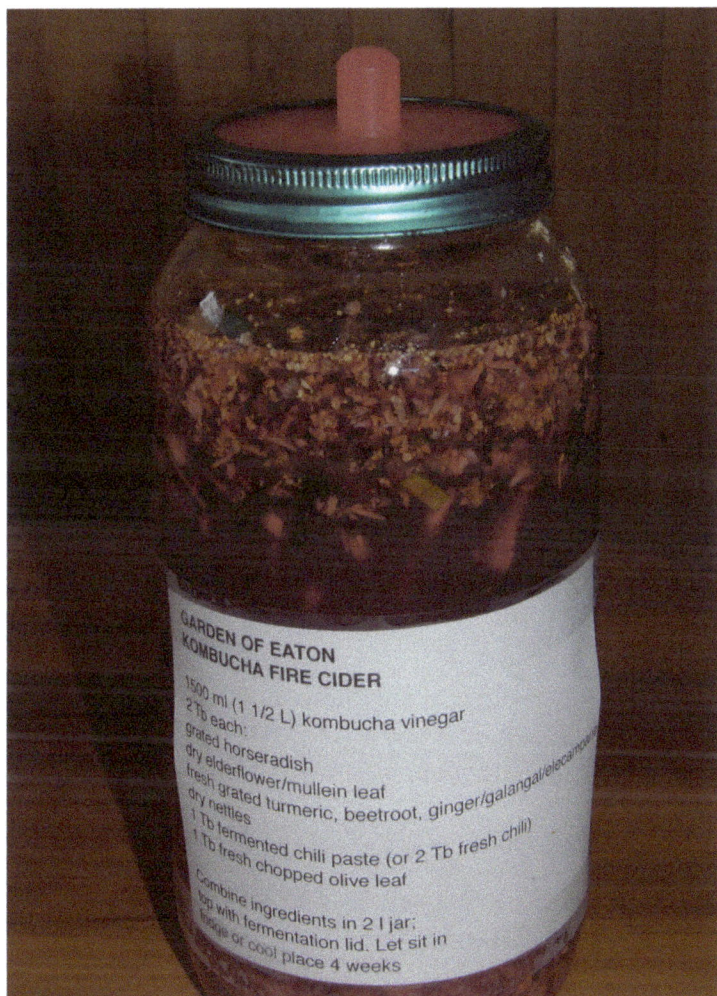

GARDEN OF EATON
KOMBUCHA FIRE CIDER

1500 ml (1 1/2 L) kombucha vinegar
2 Tb each:
grated horseradish
dry elderflower/mullein leaf
fresh grated turmeric, beetroot, ginger/galangal/elecampane
dry nettles
1 Tb fermented chili paste (or 2 Tb fresh chili)
1 Tb fresh chopped olive leaf

Combine ingredients in 2 l jar;
top with fermentation lid. Let sit in
fridge or cool place 4 weeks

Oils

Nettles can be blended with other herbs as a soothing massage oil or thickened with beeswax as an ointment or salve. I prefer to prepare my herbal oils singly and store them in brown bottles in a root cellar. For massage or salves, I then custom blend oils of choice.

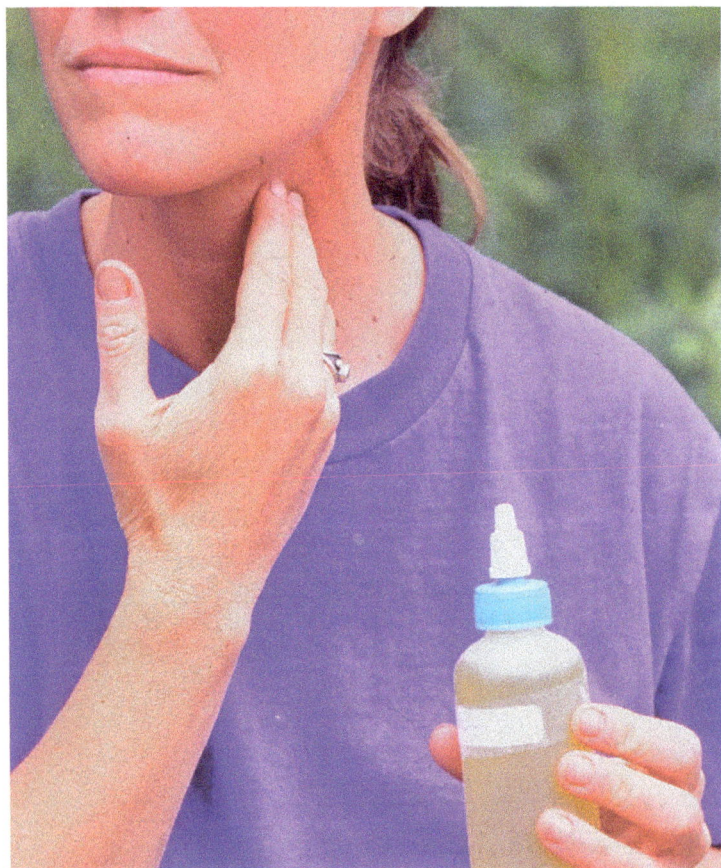

Nettle Oil

2 cups dried spring nettle leaf

1/4 cup nettle seed (if available)

3 cups extra virgin olive oil (or other oil of choice)

Combine ingredients in a 1/2 gallon jar. Place jar in a slow cooker filled with water, and heat on low for 24 to 48 hours. Strain and rebottle. Store in a colored glass jar in a root cellar.

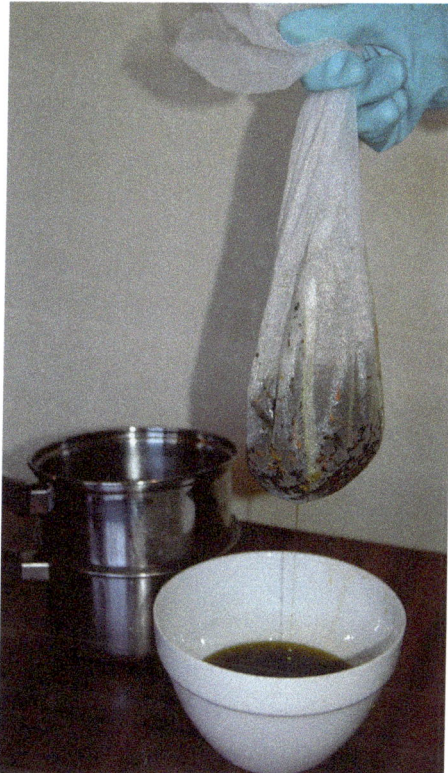

Another favorite in my kitchen combines nettle with anti-inflammatory arnica, skin regenerating calendula, and soothing dandelion flower as a "Golden Balm."

Golden Balm Massage Oil

1 cup nettle oil

1 cup arnica flower oil (*Arnica montana*)

1 cup calendula flower oil (*Calendula officinalis*)

1 cup dandelion flower oil (*Taraxacum officinalis*)

Blend oils. Scent with essential oils of choice. My favorites for massage include essential oils of fir needle, rosemary, citrus, lavender, or clove. Begin with 8 to 12 drops of essential oils, then add more, a few drops at a time, to achieve the desired aroma. I often also add flower essences, such as Bach Rescue Remedy or Alaskan flower essence. Dandelion flower essence aids in relieving muscular tension. (Flower essence sources readily available on the internet.). As a preservative, add 1/4 teaspoon vitamin E or cottonwood bud tincture (*Populus balsamifera*).

Chapter 6

Energetic Healing with Nettles

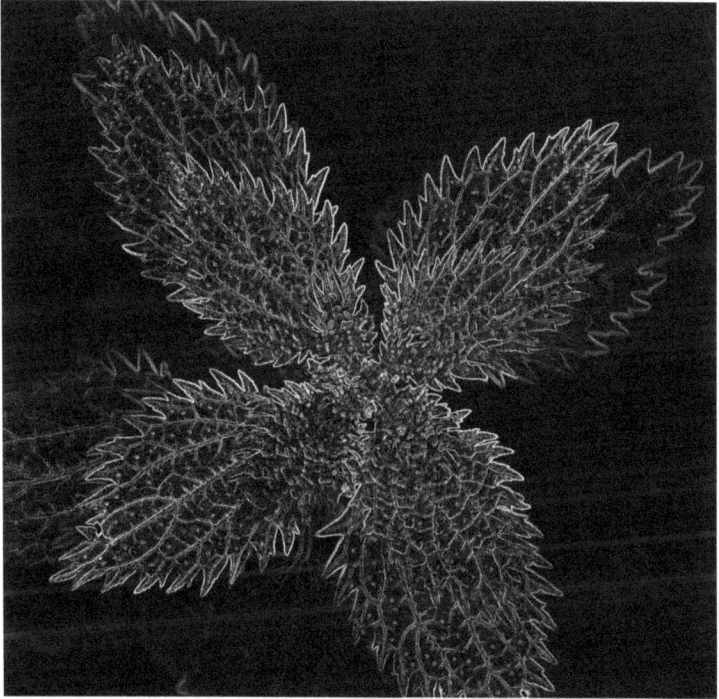

Nettle roots intertwine, linking the nettle community. Nettle also connects a human community spanning all ages and disciplines. Nettle features ln all branches of energetic medicine: western herbalism, traditional Chinese medicine, Ayurveda, and the more subtle homeopathy and flower essences.

All matter is composed of the same building blocks. But humans, animals, and plants are more than units of carbon, hydrogen, and minerals. All life infuses with energy. The ancients described this breath of life animating all beings as prana, chi, or qi. Though there are diverse systems of interpreting this energy, from quantum physics to energy medicine, what is agreed is that the life force exists.

Herbs may be viewed at the biochemistry level, categorized by the constituents they contain, enabling prediction of the biological action they will have on the human body. Clinical trials document the activity of individual constituents and measure their biological effects. Allopathy selects particular 'active ingredients' as the most important and often synthesizes or standardizes them in the laboratory. The holistic view is that major and minor compounds are all essential and act synchronistically, much like the players in an orchestra working in concert to create a symphony. Thus herbalism emphasizes the combined effect of the whole plant.

An Overview of Flower Essences

In various periods and cultures, people have collected the morning dew on plants as a healing aid. But it wasn't until the 1930s that Dr. Edward Bach in England developed the flower essence system. Discouraged by modern allopathy's bloodletting, Bach (so goes the stories I've heard) took an extended sabbatical. He noticed that sitting in various fields of flowers, or ingesting their plant dew, affected his emotional state. Since collecting morning dew was a labor-intensive and daunting process, Bach experimented with floating flowers in a bowl of pure water in direct sunlight and then taking this 'mother essence' internally. Out of this pioneering work, the Bach flower remedies were born. Today his five-flower product, Rescue Remedy, is commonly available in global pharmacies as an over-the-counter product and food supplement.

Observation of physical characteristics is one key to determining the healing qualities of a flower. Nettles, for example, cause an electrical, awakening, acupuncture-like sensation as they sting. In addition, a meditative process of deep attunement reveals properties both subtle and gross. Flower essence practitioners Steve Johnson and Jane Bell worked extensively with nettle in cocreating an essence from *Urtica* flowers. Jane Bell says: "When we were making the essence, the word dendrite kept coming to mind. Steve was led to do a funny drawing, which we later showed to a friend who was a nurse. She confirmed that Steve had indeed drawn a picture of a dendrite." (Dendrites are protoplasmic branches of the nerve cell that serve as conductors of sensation to the body of the cell.)

"Our sense," continues Jane, "was that the nettle essence might help people who have disturbances to their electrical or nervous system from accident or abuse. I have since used this essence with people who have had electric shock therapy, have been electrocuted, experience learning disabilities such as dyslexia, or experience severe nervous twitching. One summer, I attended a very demanding week-long training and took the nettle flower essence throughout. Normally I am overwhelmed by information overload, which leads to insomnia and difficulty assimilating and integrating material. With the nettle essence, I felt like the flow of information was smooth and steady."

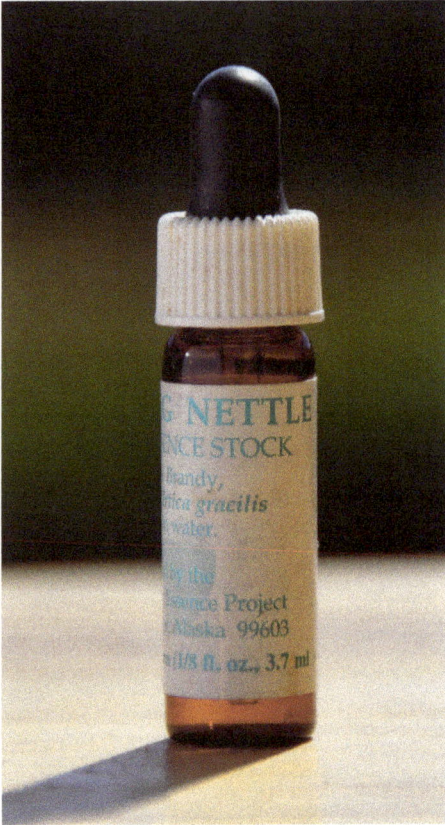

Nettles and Homeopathy

Homeopathy is a system of healing founded by the German physician Samuel Hahnemann in the late 18th century. It is based on the principle that 'like cures like.' The correct homeopathic remedy creates, in a healthy person, precisely the symptoms that the remedy cures in a sick person. Most homeopathic remedies originate in the plant, animal, and mineral kingdoms. But any natural or synthetic substance or energy may be made into a homeopathic remedy.

While in Sydney, Australia, in spring 1997, visiting herbalist Robyn Kirby, I experienced first-hand the benefits of homeopathic *Apis*, a remedy prepared from the venom of swarming bees. Many poisonous substances, including arsenic, belladonna, and water hemlock, are rendered safe for knowledgeable internal use in homeopathic form. Homeopathic preparations are repeatedly diluted and then 'succussed.' Homeopaths state that this rhythmic shaking potentizes the remedial substance and releases its etheric forces.

Medium and high potency remedies are so diluted that it is scientifically certain that not even a single molecule of the original substance remains in the medicine. In a process that cannot be explained by natural science, the higher the dilution, the more powerful the remedy becomes.

Note: When purchasing homeopathic remedies, the most commonly available form is pellets (lactose pills) infused with the homeopathic liquids. One typically takes the pellets under the tongue and allows them to dissolve. Do not attempt to substitute an herbal preparation for a homeopathic. Whereas homeopathic Arnica, for example, is safe internally because of its high dilution, internal use of an Arnica tincture could be fatal.

Homeopathic nettle is specific for skin ailments that produce symptoms similar to those of a nettle sting. *Urtica urens,* says homeopath Susan Lie-Nielsen "...seems to be one of those under-used and slightly out-of-favor remedies in the homeopathic pharmacopeia. The remedy relieves skin conditions with burning, stinging, and welts, including first-degree burns."

Testimonials regarding nettle's effectiveness in treating burns are abundantly supplied in *A Physicians' Posy* by Dorothy Shepherd. Shepherd found great success healing burned tissue with nettle homeopathic internally and nettle tincture externally. She suggests covering burns with a dressing moistened with diluted nettle tincture and reapplying fluid whenever the dressing begins to dry. "The end results," she writes, "are excellent. You get no blistering, no inflammation, and no scarring. The pain disappears within a few minutes after each application and returns when the dressing becomes dry." [26]

Homeopathic *Urtica urens* is an excellent remedy to include in any first aid kit. The potentized remedy is taken internally, and the diluted tincture is applied externally for skin conditions.

Susan Lie-Nielsen recommends *Urtica urens* for allergies, particularly for the ill effects of eating shellfish or strawberries. She reports that J. Compton-Burnet, a homeopathic physician practicing in Britain in the 19th century, found that *Urtica urens* was dramatically helpful in relieving gout symptoms. Compton-Burnet used it so often with such success that he was affectionately nicknamed Dr. Urtica.

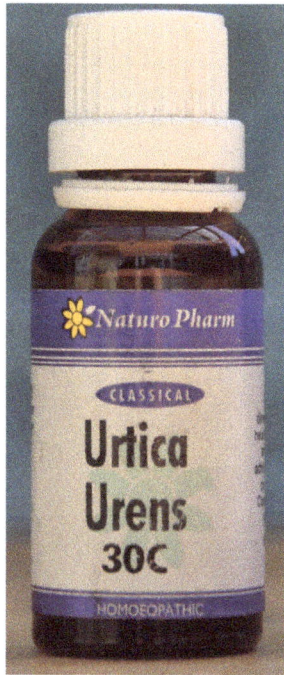

Nettle homeopathic remedy is especially indicated for rheumatism accompanied with urticaria. It is used in cases of diarrhea, combined with nettle rash or suppressed eruptions. Nettle also helps nursing mothers suffering from decreased secretion of milk for no apparent cause.

Note: There are hundreds of remedies in the homeopathic Materia Medica. Beginners often use specific classic remedies successfully in first aid situations (such as Arnica for strains and sprains, Ledum for puncture wounds, etc.). However, most conditions, especially chronic ones, require an accurate and detailed symptom picture and skillful application of the remedies. Consult a skilled homeopath for help.

The symptom picture for the use of *Urtica urens*, for example, has unique characteristics. According to homeopathic H. Reid Shaw, one feature to look for is stinging, swelling skin. Symptoms worsen after bathing, excessive exercise, and warmth. The eruption and inflammation often improve noticeably upon lying down and may reappear after rising again.

Ayurveda and Nettles

Ayurveda has been called "the mother of all healing." It originated in India over five thousand years ago and is a highly scientific system cloaked in poetic terms and metaphors. In Ayurveda's cosmic perspective, all aspects of life contain varying quantities of the essential elements (air, ether, fire, water, and earth). A skilled practitioner understands these elemental natures and balances these energies on our bodies' continuum of health. Health, as seen in Ayurveda, is a dynamic state. Health requires ever-changing adjustment to the flux of emotions, seasons, events, and physical environments. Practitioners carefully choose foods, herbs, and lifestyle routines to balance the individual.

In the Ayurvedic view, each person is born with a particular prakruti (constitution) in which one or more doshas dominate. Dosha describes energies or waste products known as Vata, Pitta, Kapha. An individual with a lot of Pitta has a combination of the elements and energies that make up Pitta (fire and water). Pitta is expressed in diverse ways, including:

- Physical characteristics (flaming red hair and fiery temper)
- Precision with details
- Redness of the skin

- A robust digestive system

- Intolerance of heat

Competitive business atmospheres or stimulating habits (such as alcohol, tobacco, and drugs) further inflame pitta energy and exacerbate inflammatory conditions.

The energies of air and ether form Vata. Vata people tend to be small-framed, mobile individuals with dry skin, cold hands and feet, and an alert, active, restless, often solitary nature. When Vata is high, the noticeable pattern is an irregularity or a consistent inconsistency. Difficulty in concentrating, constant movement, and nervous system disorders (including insomnia)

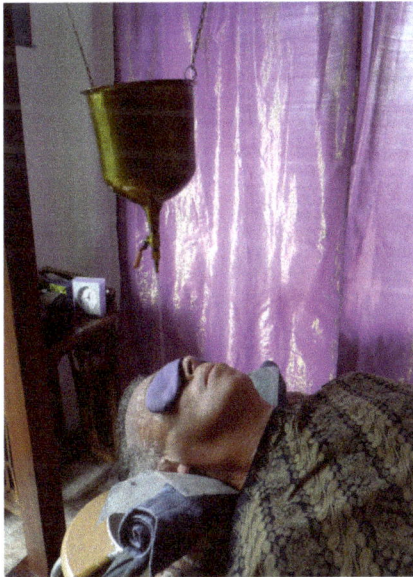

The stress-relieving Ayurvedic treatment (Shirodhara) drips medicated herbal oil onto the forehead.

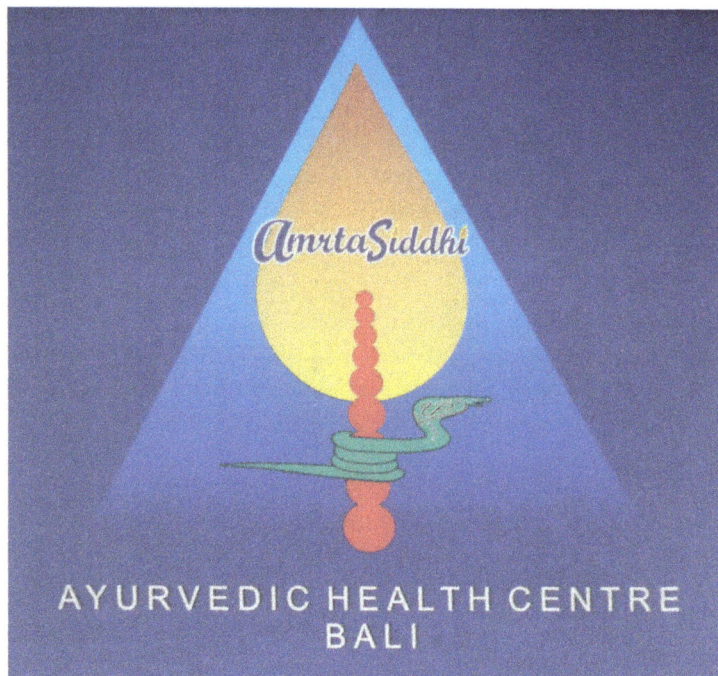

are common. Stabilizing treatment for Vatas includes the establishment of routine and more grounded cooked foods.

Kapha energy is a combination of the heavy elements of earth and water. Kapha people have a general tendency to be easy-going, larger-boned individuals who often collect books, stamps, and "stuff." When out of balance, those with high Kapha tend toward congestive disorders and lethargy. Whereas routine tends to ground the airy Vata, too much sameness keeps Kapha vegetating as couch potatoes. Kapha thrives with variety and stimulation, bright colors, aerobic exercise, frequent sex, and less frequent and lighter meals.

Ayurveda's constitution approach resolves the modern dilemma of which food is the "right" food. Because there are differing constitutions, there need to be differing diets, lifestyle routines, and herbs tailored to each. Also, the method used to prepare food or an herbal preparation affects its energetic balance.

A brief introduction such as this is far from adequate to determine one's dosha or address imbalances. Consult a skilled Ayurvedic practitioner for such purposes. This overview is merely to assist in understanding the nettle's role in the Ayurvedic system of healing.

Although there are many species of nettle in India, *Urtica dioica* is the most frequently used. In Hindi and Punjabi, the stinging nettle is called *bichu*, which means scorpion; steaming the scorpion as a vegetable benefits all doshas.

Nettle tea decreases Pitta and Kapha and increases Vata. However, nettle syrup with basil and licorice, says medical herbalist and Ayurvedic teacher Kevin Spelman, is an effective nutritive tonic for Vata dosha. Nettle potherb calms the disrupted wind, and the young spring leaves, with their laxative effect, benefit the dry Vata nature. Nesto (nettle pesto) is also an excellent food for the deficient Vata. Spelman adds:

"The experience of nettles in the field reminds one of cellular nutrition, the blood vessels of the body, the cilia of the respiratory tract, and the villi of the gastrointestinal tract. Consider its use for those who are depleted and exhausted at a core level. This could include those who are convalescing, malnourished, or undergoing or recovering from chemotherapy or radiation therapies. Steamed nettles as a food or taken as a syrup provide excellent therapy for these conditions."

New research shows that the gut binds large amounts of serotonin, and one of the nettle's constituents is serotonin. Thus nettles may help to improve mood as well as the digestive tract. Perhaps nettles can be especially useful in those inflammatory gastrointestinal conditions that have a strong emotional component, such as irritable bowel syndrome and gastrointestinal ulcers.

In Ayurvedic practice, yet another tissue that nettle treats is the skin.

Nettle tincture applied topically (diluted 1:1 with water) effectively treats burns both from the sun and heat and rashes (even the inflammation from nettle itself) and other red-hot inflammatory conditions.

As an Indian folk remedy, nettle is used for renal complaints and hemorrhages. Nettle is categorized as astringent, diuretic, and a significant hemostatic. Use includes:

catarrh (mucous membrane inflammation)

leukorrhea (excess vaginal or cervical mucus)

bronchial hemorrhage, blood-spitting

uterine hemorrhage

nephritis (kidney inflammation)

hematuria (blood in the urine)

menorrhagia (excessive menstrual bleeding).

Another species, *U. parviflora*, has been given to reduce fevers.

In Ayurvedic terms, the energetics of nettles Are:

Rasa (taste): leaf: astringent, sweet; root: sweet, astringent

Virya (energy): leaf and root: cool

Gunas (qualities): light and dry

Vipaka (systemic effect): leaf and root: sweet, heavy

Traditional Chinese Medicine

Traditional Chinese Medicine (TCM) is another highly developed and respected system of healing. The Chinese five-element system classifies these elements as water, earth, fire, wood, and metal. The water element is associated with the kidney and bladder, the earth with stomach and spleen-pancreas, fire with heart (as well as the pericardium and small intestine), metal with large intestine and lungs, and wood with liver and gall bladder.

In the Chinese system, herbs and foods are characterized by their nature, flavor, direction, and the organs/meridians they affect. The nature of an herb has to do with the quality of heat or coolness that the herb generates. (Contrast the cooling effect of nettles and mint to the stimulating warmth of dry ginger or Mexican chilies). Flavor is not just something that makes food taste good; it is a therapeutic tool in energetic medicine.

Nettle's flavor, according to TCM, is salty/sweet, affecting both fluid balance and organ tonification. Its astringency contracts tissues, lessening excess secretions.

TCM also views herbs from a directional perspective. "Lighter herbs, like herbs and flowers," writes TCM practitioner Michael Tierra, "tend to float and ascend, making them useful for more acute and surface diseases, such as colds, flu, and inflammations. Heavier herbs such as barks, seeds, and roots, descend and sink and are more effective in treating deeper, more chronic diseases." [27]

Shoshanna Sadow of the Alaska Center for Traditional Medicine tested my pulses before and after ingestion of nettle leaf infusion and root decoction. She noted that the leaf infusion soothed or harmonized my pulse's superficial aspect (making it less floating and more even). The leaf tea also stimulated circulation to the yang organs (large intestine, stomach, gall bladder, urinary bladder, and small intestine/triple burner). A distinct shift occurred when I ingested nettle root decoction. The substance of the pulse changed; the yin pulses "rooted" and strengthened. The yin pulses are associated with the deeper internal yin organs (kidney, spleen, liver, lung, and heart/pericardium).

According to Sadow, the functions of nettles are fivefold in TCM:

1. Nettle lowers heat (as in infections) and congestion in the kidney and urinary bladder and stomach, spleen, and liver.

2. Nettle clears dampness and phlegm in the lungs (especially "hot," i.e., yellow or green mucus). It significantly benefits heat-type asthma, like that characterized by a red face, rapid heavy breathing, yellow or sticky mucus, and body heat (which may be indicated by dry or hard stools and scanty urine).

3. Nettle clears damp-heat from the large intestine. Consider nettle in inflammatory "itis" diseases (such as diverticulitis). Diarrhea may indicate the presence of toxins in combination with dampness and heat. Symptoms may include burning water diarrhea, often with blood or mucus, a red tongue with a greasy, yellow coating, and a slippery pulse. Herpes, boils, and HIV also indicates damp heat.

4. Nettle cools hot blood. A red tongue, red skin eruptions, fever, thirst, fast pulse, and bright red blood indicate "hot blood" to a TCM practitioner. Heat and fire toxins penetrating the blood level are said to agitate the blood and increase the possibility of reckless blood (hemorrhage). Thus nettle is used to treat bleeding of the lungs, nose, gastrointestinal tract, kidneys, and urinary bladder.

5. Nettle tonifies the blood, including the liver blood as well as the hair (called the "glory of the blood" in TCM). Nettle root also tonifies kidney jing (our deep level constitutional essence). Jing aids in determining the major cycles in our life and encompasses both yin and yang. Nettle is also said to build the "Wei Qi," the protective Qi (chi) or energy of the body, thus increasing disease resistance.

Readers Notes

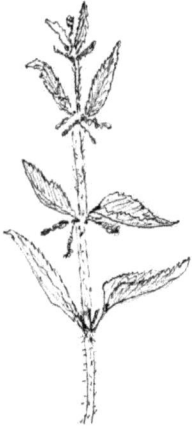

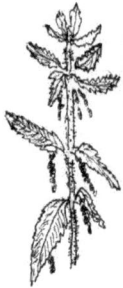

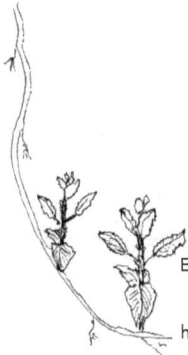

E-mail your new recipes and nettle experiences to:
athomewithjanice@gmail.com
for potential inclusion in the blog:
https://www.athomewithjaniceschofieldeaton.com

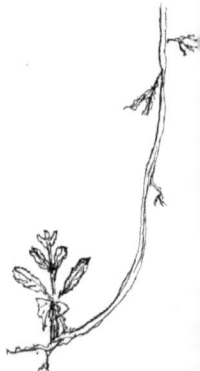

Chapter 7

Nettles For Animal Health

For immunity reasons, orphan lambs require a feed of colostrum (from milk obtained from a ewe who has lambed in the past twenty-four hours). After that period, transition to milk powder. Instead of mixing milk powder into plain water, I often substituted nettle tea for the water. The nettles give the lambs an extra nutritional boost. (Make sure the water or tea used is 108-109 F (42-43 C), slightly warmer than lamb's average body temperature.

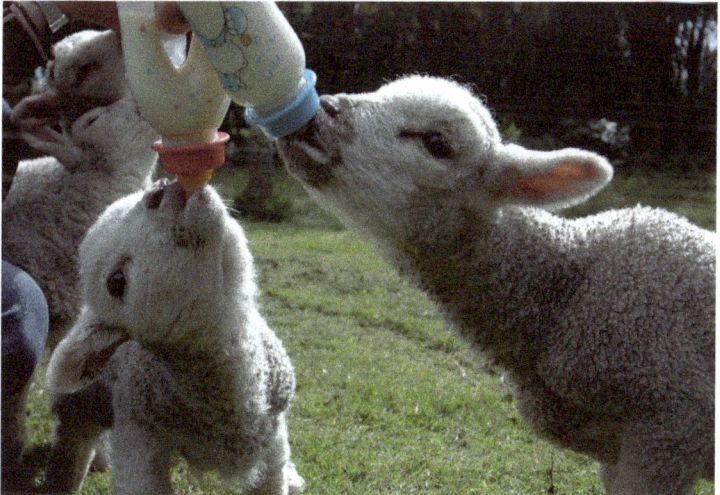

Farmers generally feed orphan lambs twice daily. My flexible home schedule allows frequent feeds, a method that more closely mimics the natural state (lambs receive small regular meals from their mothers).

According to the Richmond New Zealand Vet Centre, "New lambs need around 15 percent of body weight in milk over 24 hours, but in 6-8 feeds, e.g., a 3 kg lamb (this is an average size) needs 300-450 ml of milk per 24 hrs, but only 50-75 ml per feed. The lamb will still appear hungry after this! Never feed the lamb until its stomach starts to bulge or until it doesn't want any more. Gradually increase the amount fed as the lamb grows. At 3 weeks old, 4 feeds of 250mls each per day should be about right. Lambs should have milk until about 12 to 14 weeks old."

I know from personal experience that overfeeding lambs can trigger abomasal bloat (abdominal swelling) and potential death.

(Cracked teats that flow milk too quickly can also stimulate bloat.) New Zealand's Franklin Vets advocate yoghurtised milk at every feed as bloat prevention. (Check their website https://franklinvets.co.nz for complete directions and additional tips for successful orphan lamb rearing.)

Nettles and Poultry

Greek herbalist-author Juliet de Bairacli Levy touted nettle seed as a fattener for poultry. Juliet boiled older leaves into a mash with cereals, and fed very young raw leaves, cut small, into poultry feed. I use 5-bladed kitchen scissors to snip newly emerging nettles into the breakfast rations for the chickens. Add cooked nettles into winter mash.

Crushed leaves added to chicken and duck feed are reported to enhance egg-laying and prevent and cure coccidiosis (a parasitic protozoan) in baby chicks. Studies by Kolouset et al.

demonstrated 22 to 23 percent weight gain in nettle-fed chicks; hemoglobin content increased 5 percent. [28]

Ana Herman, the chief product strategist of Farmeron, adds that "...the addition of nettles in poultry feeding can increase protein intake by 15-20% and vitamin intake by 60-70% while reducing the need for green food by 30%."

Nutritious herbs, like wilted nettle and plantain leaves, reports Weston A. Price Foundation author Jen Allbriton, "boost egg production and yolk hue." Though chicken farmers often feed just pellets and grains to their hens, they are omnivores and designed to consume a wide diversity of insects, worms, grasses, and herbs.

Nepal researchers noted that nettles fed to chickens improved egg productivity and immunity.

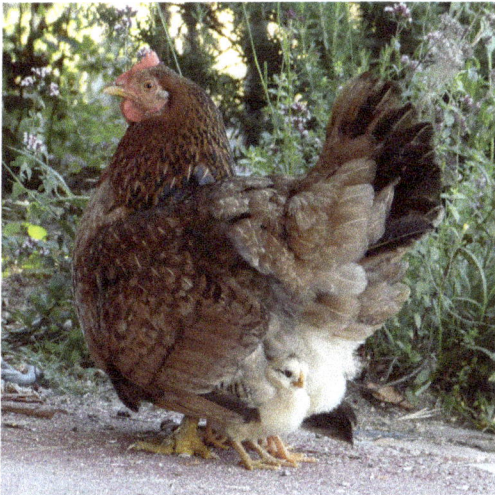

Happy Hens Feed Blend

(organic, if available)

10 pounds (4.5 kg) wheat

2.2 pounds (1 kg) cracked corn (blue or yellow)

2.2 pounds (1 kg) hulled barley

2.2 pounds (1 kg) oats

2.2 pounds (1 kg) sesame seeds (brown or black)

2.2 pounds (1 kg) sunflower seeds

1/2 pound (.22 kg) nettle seed

1/2 pound (.22 kg) chia

1/2 pound (.22 kg) dried dulse or kelp flakes

Nettles and Budgerigars (Parakeets) and Parrots

I follow Birds Online's advice and freeze nettle tips with seeds as supplementary feed for my budgies. Freezing deactivates the sting. Alternately, you can feed the fresh seeding tips after

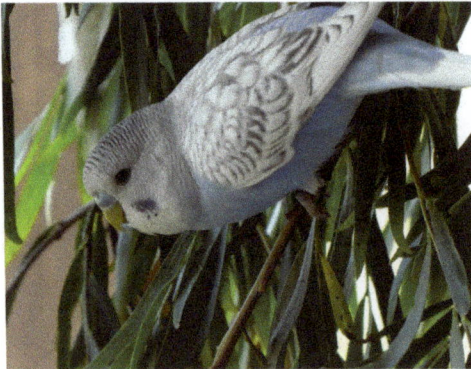

blanching in water. Nettle leaf is an ingredient in several commercial pellets for feeding birds.

Nettles and Dogs and Cats

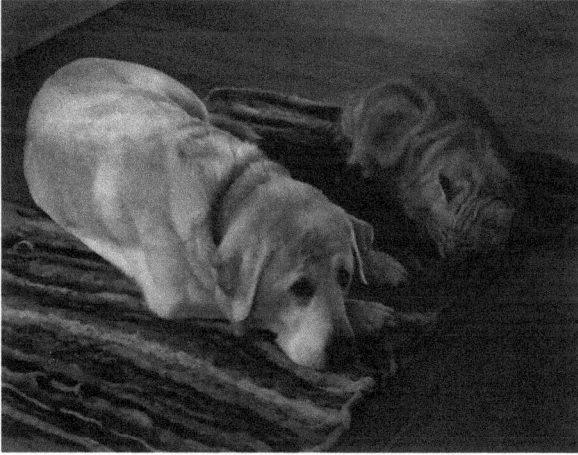

Add powdered dry nettles, or cooked fresh nettles, to your dog's feed as a nutritional supplement. Holistic veterinarian Dr. Jodie Gruenstern also recommends cooled nettle leaf tea " as a coat or even eye rinse for itchy skin or itchy eyes." (Be aware that pets can be harmed if they stumble into a nettle patch.)

Cats also thrive with dry nettle added to their cat food. Oregon vet Keith Weingardt advises 1/3 teaspoon of nettle per pound of cat food (and ½ teaspoon dry nettle per pound of dog food).

Nettles and Other Livestock

Nettles, reports Greek herbalist Juliet de Bairacli Levy, increases milk production in lactating animals and decreases round and threadworms (via a drench of nettles boiled in whey). Pigs thrive with boiled nettles added to their feed.

Feed boiled or dried nettles to pigs. A Polish research paper documented that meat from pigs fed nettle had higher protein and less fat. Supplementing their diet with nettles "...increased the lightness of meat and stabilized meat color for 6 months of storage at -20°C. Moreover, it slightly improved meat oxidative stability during frozen storage." [29]

The following YouTube video shows a Ukrainian farmer using a chaff cutter to chop nettles for feeding his pigs and poultry: https://youtu.be/PqaZ5i_5U_g.

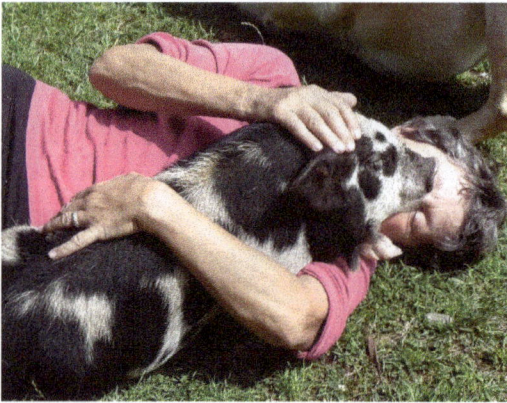

In Successful Farming's Farmeron Lesson on feeding cattle, they reported that cows fed hay or silage containing nettle "...show a significant increase in milk production and increase in milk fat – up to 15-20%." Alaskan Mairiis Kilcher, in personal communication, noted that her homesteading family knew precisely when the cows had been grazing on spring nettles. Their milk became yellowish, creamy, indescribably delicious, and energizing.

Nettles and Horses

Nettle leaf and seeds are a fantastic supplement to add to winter mash for horses, And dry nettles, added to hay, rival cottonseed meal in protein content. Feed freely to horses, as well as cattle, goats, and rabbits. Grass hay studies (containing nettles) by Kolouset et al. showed nettle's organic and mineral nutrients higher than all hays, including alfalfa, and the amount of bound amino acids twice as high as alfalfa and clover." [30]

In Germany, clinical trials using nettles in treating racehorses with coughs and nasal mucus were deemed positive.

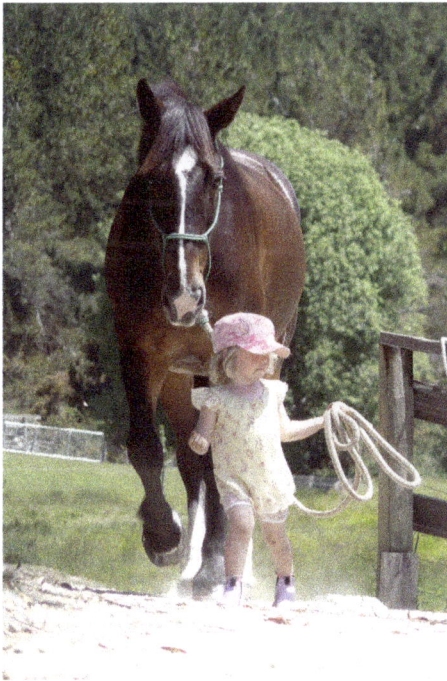

Riley Nelson-Knauf leading Clyde

Nettle leaf, writes Bruce Burnet, author of *HerbWise: Growing, Cooking, Wellbeing*, supplies "albuminoid, an excellent conditioning protein that gives the animals a sleek coat."

Holistic veterinary medicine pioneer, the late Juliet de Baracli Levy, advocated mixing fresh spring nettle juice with nettle seed and using it internally and externally to encourage "beautiful dappling and shine on horses." She found that the seed inspired appetite and made equines more spirited. [31]

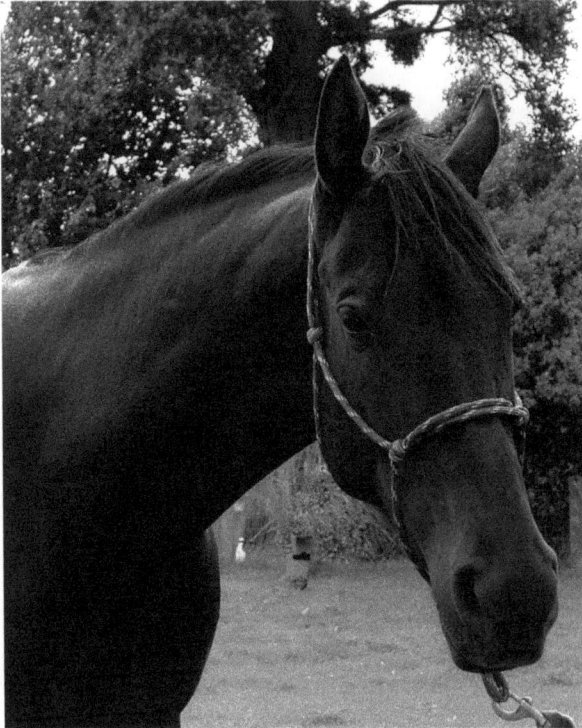

Crafty horse traders, reported Suzanne Fischer-Rizzi, used nettle seeds in transforming old or debilitated animals into saleable items. Finnish herbalist Henriette Kress adds additional details in her blog: "Back in the 1800s, dishonest horse peddlers in Germany, Hungary, and Ireland (and probably other places) used to give 1-2 handfuls of nettle seed a day to horses for about 2 weeks before they took them to market. This gave the horses shiny pelts and a youthful appearance and brought a handsome price." The vim and vigor dissipated when the new owners failed to feed nettle seed.

Henriette further describes a German doctor working in a home for the elderly who decided to mimic the horse trader's secret. He had the nurses give 1-2 tablespoons of dried nettle seed a day to all the inmates. "His patients got interested in life again, got the energy to do things, and some of them even got some fire back into their libido. Ever since I read about that German doc, I've used nettle seeds for run-down, overly tired, burned-out, or just bone-weary people -- folks who would do things if they just had the energy for it. [32]

Nettle seeds are adaptogenic, helping animals (and humans) relieve stress. They are a vitamin tonic containing nutrients from A to zinc. They strengthen the adrenals and tonify all organ systems—a definite plus for man and beast.

Readers Notes

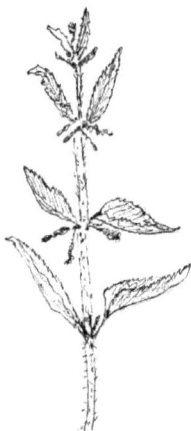

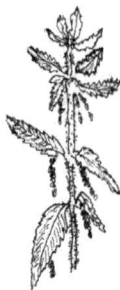

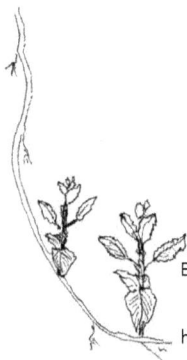

E-mail your new recipes and nettle experiences to:
athomewithjanice@gmail.com
for potential inclusion in the blog:
https://www.athomewithjaniceschofieldeaton.com

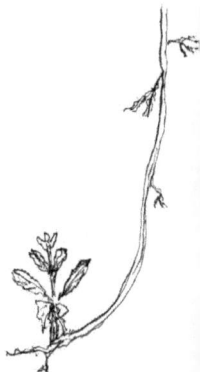

Chapter 8

Nettles, The Garden, and Soil Nutrition

My love affair with nettles began with the volunteer seedlings at the historic homestead cabin where I resided during my first Alaskan year.

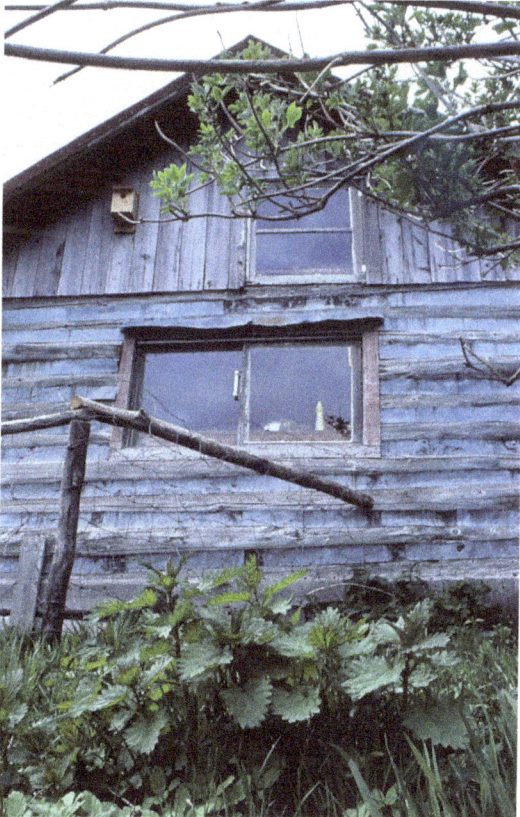

Three decades later, I revisited the Swift Creek cabin to continue the spring tradition of feasting on the gourmet greens.

Nettles are the vegetable I absolutely "most miss" when absent on a property. Their flavor, nutrient density, and adaptability make them my number one edible and tonic herb.

When I moved to my New Zealand property, nettles were sorely absent. I obtained my first European nettle seedlings from a booth at a Steiner School Fair. Other than nettles gifted to local herb and butterfly (see chapter 10) enthusiasts, my nettles have remained 'at home' Each year, my patch provides abundant opportunities to feed ourselves, our animals, and our soil.

Another nettle, the dwarf *Urtica urens*, 'hitchhiked' to our property when we imported hops compost. Since I prefer eating the larger European variety, I till dwarf nettle back into the soil to feed my compost heap.

Cultivation

If you lack a source of seedlings, you can cultivate nettle from seed (check the internet for a source near you). Peter Borchard of Companion Plants recommends starting seeds in spring or fall. He sows his seed in well-drained commercial potting soil, covers the small seeds very lightly, and keeps them warm and moist. Seedlings should appear within a fortnight.

Be certain that you plant your nettles in an appropriate area, as their trailing rhizomes (underground stems) DO trail. Be aware that your patch can expand three feet (a meter) in a year. You may wish to restrict nettles with a physical barrier (as is commonly done with mints.) Another option is to plant them in a large container.

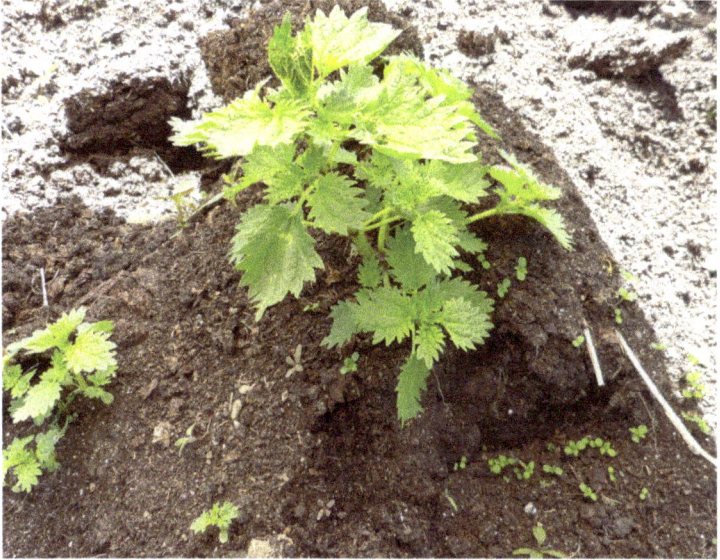

Companion Planting

Nettles are a popular companion plant for tomatoes, and tomatoes store well in a root cellar packed in dry nettle leaves. According to the Old Farmer's Almanac, "plants grown in the presence of stinging nettle display exceptional vigor and resist spoiling."

Helen Philbrick and Richard Gregg, authors of *Companion Plants and How to Use Them*, state that "Nettles change the chemical process of neighboring crops."

Grown as a companion plant, add Philbrick and Gregg, nettle "increased the content of essential oil up to 20% in valerian, over 80% in *Angelica archangelica*, 10 to 20% in marjoram, 10% in sage, and 10% in peppermint." Growers alternate three rows of aromatic herbs (such as mint, chamomile, and valerian) with one row of nettles to increase essential oils 10 to 20 percent.

Composting with Nettles

In the wild, nettles are an indicator of good soil with abundant nitrogen. Nettles themselves enrich the soil and contribute to humus formation. In a personal experiment, Alaskan Mairiis Kilcher found that flowers planted in pots containing soil dug from nettle-rich areas grew plants twice the size of the controls.

Fresh or dry nettle is an invaluable addition to compost. Compost is nutrient-rich matter formed by layering green matter (vegetable and fruit scraps, leftover garden materials), brown carbon-rich matter (leaves, straw, sawdust), and animal manures. (Avoid adding roots unless the compost pile is extremely hot.)

Biodynamic Preparation 504 is made from stinging nettle buried underground in an earthenware container and left to break down for a year. Following biodynamic principles, harvest nettles early in the day, between dawn and noon. (This timing coincides with the height of photosynthesis and the peak of the plant's vitality for the above-ground parts.) Dig a hole approximately one yard (meter) long and one and a half feet (.45 meter) deep. In the bottom of the hole, spread a handful of peat moss and then begin laying in the cut nettles. Top with sphagnum moss and then cover with earth. Ensure the dimensions of the hole are well marked so that you can find your BD504 a year later when you dig up your nettle. Add a small amount of the finished BD504 to compost to stimulate soil health and nutrition.

The biodynamic quick-return method of compost-making eliminates the demands of turning the compost manually as the following "herbal activator" stimulates the fermentation process:

Biodynamic Herbal Activator

1 part each:

stinging nettle (*Urtica* species)

yarrow (*Achillea millefolium*)

dandelion (*Taraxacum officinale*)

chamomile (*Matricaria recutita*)

valerian (*Valeriana officinalis*)

oak bark (*Quercus* species)

Australian author Gail Stern recommends gathering the herbs early in the morning and crushing them separately after drying. Mix equal parts in a container. Combine 1 part dry herb blend with 20 parts rainwater and shake well. Allow the 'tea' to rest for 24 hours.

Then poke holes in the compost heap every foot with a 2-inch (5 cm) diameter stick and pour 3 inches (7.5 cm) of herbal activator into every hole. Cover the pile with soil and leave for one month; after which time the compost should be rich, black, and crumbly. [33]

Plant Fertilizer and Aphid Spray

Prepare a fermented plant fertilizer by placing freshly harvested nettles in a plastic container. Cover a generous pile of nettles with fresh water and a lid and allow it to stand outdoors, well away from your house, for about two weeks. Finnish herbalist Henriette Kress comments that with this method, "everything but the seeds have dissolved, and it stinks to high heaven. Add nine parts fresh water to one part nettle water and use as a fertilizer." Doing this with older plants is an excellent way to get more nettles as the seeds will sprout. To avoid 'spreading,' use young plants.

Brew a quicker (and non-odorous) plant tea by infusing nettles for three days. Fill a bucket with nettle greens and cover with water. Pour through a sieve; discard the spent nettles in the compost pile. Dilute with three parts of freshwater. I've experienced success feeding this to plants to ease transplanting shock. You can also place this tea in a spritzer bottle as a spray for aphids; add a few drops of a non-toxic soap to increase adherence to the leaves.

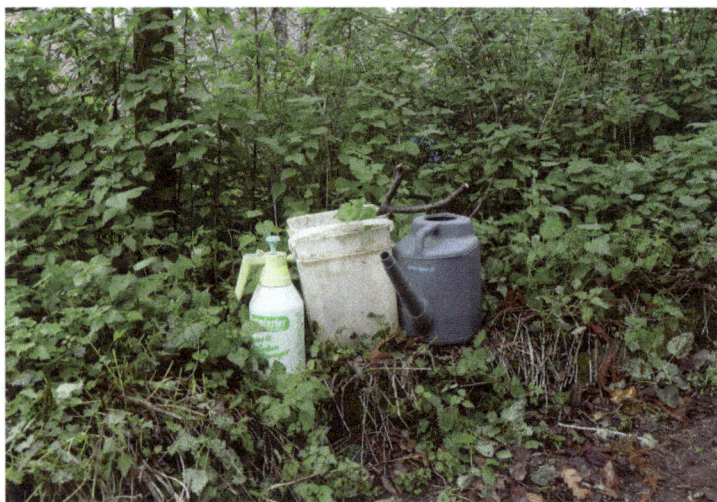

Another option is to use fresh-pressed nettle juice (use a wheat-grass juicer) as a compost additive. Or dilute 20:1 as an insect spray or plant-grow fertilizer. For molds and mildew in the greenhouse, combine nettle juice with fireweed (*Epilobium angustifolium*) or other anti-fungal herbs, or Neem oil.

Following is an Irish recipe for Nettle brew by James Kilkelly of www.gardenplansireland.co. Preparation requires first equipping yourself with: strong gloves, long-sleeved clothing, sharp garden clippers, and a canvas or hessian bag. Fill your sack with a kilo (2.2 pounds) of chopped, non-flowering nettles. Place in a barrel, top with 20 liters (quarts) water, weigh down with rocks or bricks and cover.

Allow the mixture to brew for a month; then dilute 10 parts water to 1 part nettle brew, and water freely around the base of your plants.

Leave the mix to brew for about three or four weeks before you consider applying it. When the time comes, mix it in your watering can at a rate of 10 parts water to 1 part nettle brew, then water liberally around your plants.

Readers Notes

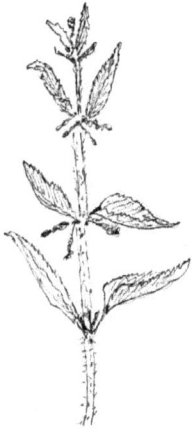

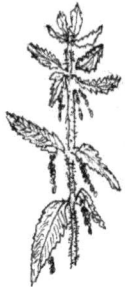

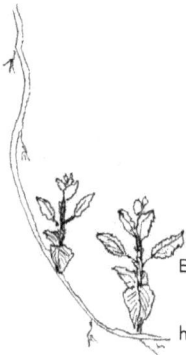

E-mail your new recipes and nettle experiences to:
athomewithjanice@gmail.com
for potential inclusion in the blog:
https://www.athomewithjaniceschofieldeaton.com

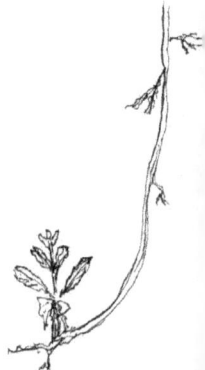

Chapter 9

Nettles, Earth Health, and Butterflies

The canary is to the coal mine as the butterfly is to the planet- an environmental health indicator. Butterflies and bees are floral pollinators, crucial to crop health and productivity. Rampant development, deforestation, and pesticides decimate their populations.

Various butterflies (including the red admiral, peacock, and comma) use nettle plants as a repository for eggs and a nursery for their emerging caterpillars. On Alaska's Kenai Peninsula, caterpillars of the black and gold Milbert's tortoiseshell butterfly (*Aglais milberti*) feed solely on stinging nettle. The caterpillars enthusiastically browse the nettle leaves. "At first, the young

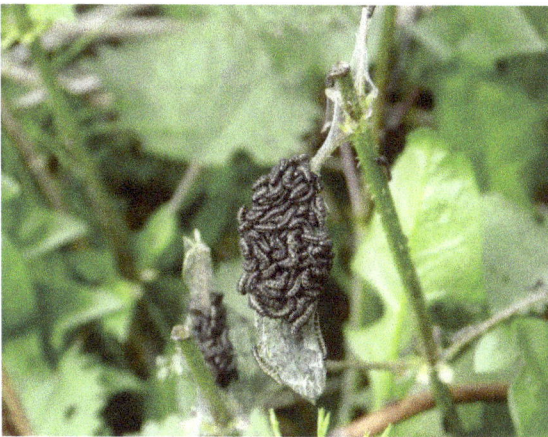

Nettle caterpillars in Alaska, photo by Ellen Vande Visse

caterpillars feed together within a loose tent made of silk threads," writes wildlife ecologist Ed Berg. "As they grow in size, the caterpillars disperse on their food plant and eventually make cocoons among the leaves. The bristle-covered caterpillar of the red admiral butterfly (*Vanessa atalanta*), which is black with red bands and white spots, also feeds on nettles in Interior Alaska. [34]

Berg notes that nettles also provide seeds for birds. Birds forage both on the caterpillars and on aphids that also live on nettles.

According to the Moths and Butterflies of New Zealand Trust, the red admiral butterfly, *Bassaris gonerilla* (formerly *Vanessa gonerilla* and called *kahukura* by the Maori), is endemic to New Zealand. This species is not found naturally anywhere else in the world. (Check their website for fascinating butterfly facts, inspiring projects, and their Beginner's Guide to Nettles.) [35]

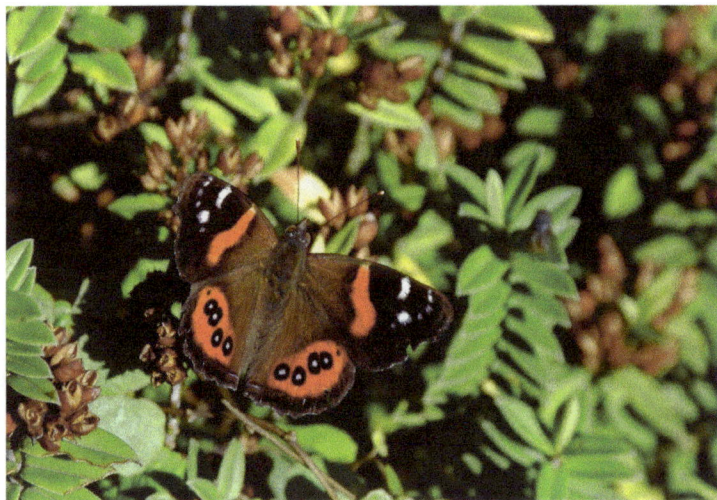

In New Zealand, red admiral numbers were common a century ago. Their population plummeted after New Zealand deliberately imported parasitic wasps (*Pteromalus puparum*) from England in 1933 to control the cabbage white butterfly. Declines in host plant availability also contributed to a dwindling admiral population.

The NZ red Admiral caterpillar's preferred food is the ferocious-to-humans `(ongaonga or tree nettle). (This nettle has killed at least one man with its venomous stings but is safe fodder for the butterflies.)

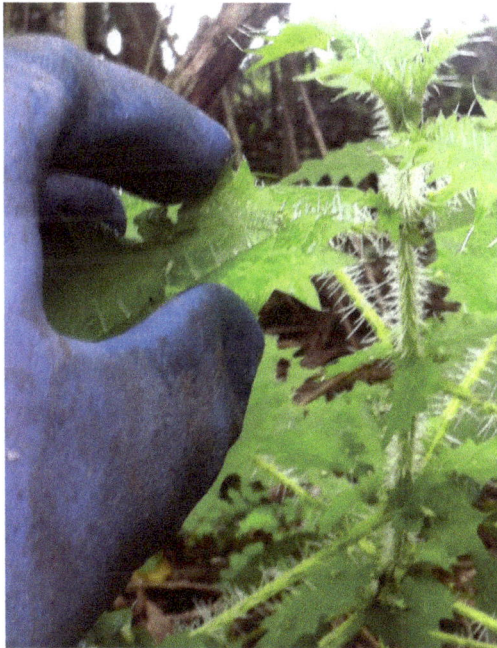

NZ tree nettle, *Urtica ferox*

The caterpillars feed on all nettles, both introduced and native, including scrub nettle (*Urtica incisa*), rough nettle (*Urtica aspera*), and dwarf nettle (*Urtica urens*).

Nettles are also hosts for the Australasian yellow admiral Butterflies.

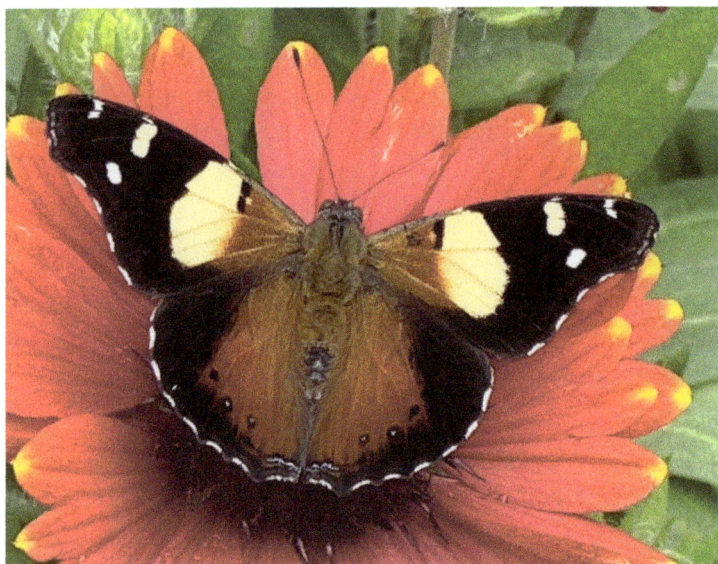

New Zealand Yellow Admiral butterfly, photo courtesy Jacqui Knight

Kiwi butterfly lover, the late Peter Brennan, raised over 360 yellow admiral butterflies in a single year. Brennan planted nettles in his Sandspit garden and in pots. "The pots," he'd written, "can be moved under mosquito netting to protect caterpillars and chrysalis from predatory wasps." [36] To learn more about how to grow a nettle butterfly garden and protect your pupa from being parasitized by wasps, etc., view the Graeme Hill

Youtube: https://youtu.be/SJpBNMGgzQs. Hill raises 150-200 native butterflies each year.

The Oratia New Zealand Native Plant nursery, reported Stuff online news, sold three species of native nettles. Interest in nettles for butterfly gardening was so strong that they experienced a tenfold increase in sales- from 20 plants a year to around 200. Oratia Nursery, unfortunately, is now closed, but seeds and plants of other stinging nettles are frequently available at https://www.nzbutterflies.org.nz/items-for-sale/seeds/

In Auckland, New Zealand, Rob Jones of Forest & Bird has worked with the Auckland Council to reintroduce nettles and other butterfly plants to parks to boost butterfly numbers and increase biodiversity. Check out their "How To" guide for attracting native butterflies to your garden. [37]

Jones reports that the caterpillars of NZ red admiral butterflies eat most native and non-native nettles, but that yellow admirals prefer natives. However, Jacqui Knight of the Moth and Butterflies Trust has observed that both admiral species lay eggs on whatever nettles you have.

Note: Be aware that in Otago, New Zealand, European nettle is considered a pest plant and restricted from being distributed or grown.

New Zealand butterflies nectar heavily on the native hebe and rata. Swan plants (sold in plant nurseries) are host plants of monarch butterflies (*Danaus plexippus*). According to the online encyclopedia Te Ara, "The Monarch was first recorded in New Zealand in 1873, having island-hopped its way across the Pacific Ocean from North America." This behavior is contrary to most insects, which come from the opposite direction, borne on Australia's strong westerly winds. [38]

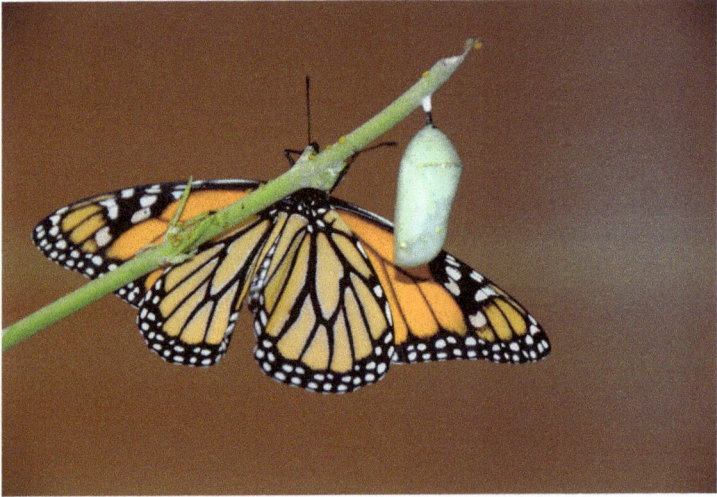

Above is one of the three dozen monarchs I raised in my home on a spare table. Watching their life cycle from egg to butterfly emerging from the chrysalis provided hours of entertainment.

Since the 1940s, five wasp species were introduced to NZ, both deliberately (for cabbage butterfly control) and accidentally. British Broadcasting Corporation praises wasps for their role in the pollination of crops and insect control. The BBC describes them as "voracious and ecologically important predators." But this skill is terrible news for treasured NZ butterflies like the native admirals. Are wasps affecting butterflies on your property? Following is a photo-illustrated source guide to wasp identification: https://www.nzbutterflies.org.nz/wp-content/uploads/2020/02/Predatory-wasps.pdf

To safeguard your butterflies from wasps, the Moths and Butterflies of NZ Trust advocate three options:

1. Grow your butterfly host plants in pots so that you can move them to less wasp-prone locations. For example: close to bushes, so they can be camouflaged by other plants. (Solitary swan plants, for example, are a siren call for wasps.)

2. Grow them under a cover, such as a mosquito net. (Or check an op shop for an old net curtain).

3. Purchase a 'caterpillar castle'. One source is https://www.nzbutterflies.org.nz/items-for-sale/caterpillar-castles/.

In regards to growing native nettles for hosting butterflies, Forest and Bird, in its How-To guide referenced earlier reports:

"All of these nettles grow best in damp, semi-shady areas and loamy, nitrogen-rich soil. Chicken-coops, or farms often provide the high-nitrogen levels they need, so they're commonly found around these areas. Topdressing the nettles with sheep pellets from a nursery helps to create this high nutrient environment. Admirals locate nettles by following the trail of oils that they produce. For this reason, it is best to plant a patch of nettles (~4m2 is a good size) that is free of any other butterfly plants because scents of other plants can overpower the volatile cues the butterflies follow."

Be sure to wear gloves and long-sleeve shirts when working around the butterfly nettle patch.

In the United Kingdom, the CONE organization promotes environmental projects, including wildlife havens, strawbale swallow barns, and nettle gardens for butterflies. UK butterfly species that utilize nettle plants to feed their larvae include: the brush-footed red admiral (*Vanessa atalanta*), small tortoiseshell (*Aglais urticae*), peacock (*Inachis io*), and comma (*Polygonia c-album*).

CONE promotes an annual May event titled: Be Nice to Nettles Week. Project Co-ordinator Phil Castiaux states: "I think it is important to recognize the value of nettles and the role that these and other weeds play in the wider environment. I hope National Be Nice to be Nettles Week goes some way towards improving the image of the nettle." Additional United Kingdom events include:

- Nettle Appreciation Day at Nowton Park in Bury St Edmunds.

- Big Nature Day at the Natural History Museum, London (with a walk along the Nettle Trail in the Museum's Wildlife Garden).

- Be Nice to Nettles at Woodland's Farm.

Within Buckingham Palace gardens, says head gardener Mark Lane: "nettles play an important role in the wildlife habitat areas providing a valuable food source for caterpillars." [39]

The following are but a few of the economic and ecological benefits highlighted in "*Urtica* spp.: Ordinary Plants with Extraordinary Properties, published in *Molecules* Journal. [40]

Nettles:

- Improve soils over-fertilized with nitrogen and phosphate.

- Promote local flora and fauna biodiversity.

- Support over 40 species of insects.

- Reduce heavy metal content in the soil.

- Produce high-quality agricultural raw materials for dyeing, textile, and energy sectors.

The simple act of cultivating nettles is a healing boon for a stressed planet. Want to 'be greener?' Grow nettles!

Readers Notes

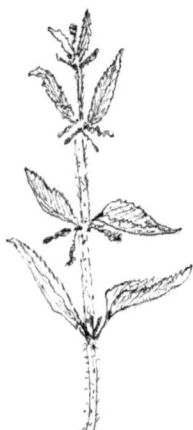

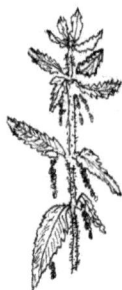

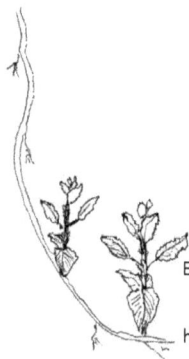

E-mail your new recipes and nettle experiences to:
athomewithjanice@gmail.com
for potential inclusion in the blog:
https://www.athomewithjaniceschofieldeaton.com

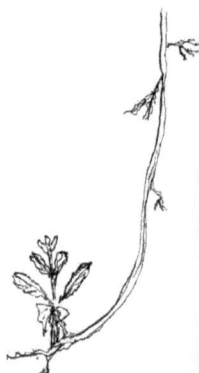

Chapter 10

Nettle Games, Songs, Folklore, and Fiber

The Scottish have such reverence for nettles that they have immortalized them in song. In the ancient Scottish tune, following, the words 'cowe' and 'stoo' mean to "cut, crop or harvest," and 'kail' is an old name for nettle potherb. Make up your own melody and sing this ancient verse in the shower, or better yet, in the nettle patch as you cowe the nettle.

Cowe the Nettle [41]

Gin ye be for lang kail,
Cowe the nettle, stoo the nettle,
Gin ye be for lang kail,
Cowe the nettle early.

Cowe it laich, cowe it sune,
Cowe it in the month o' June;
Stoo it ere it's in the bloom,
Cowe the nettle early.

Cowe it by the old wa's,
Cowe it where the sun ne'er fa's,
Stoo it when the day daws,
Cowe the nettle early.

Dried nettle, sprinkled around a room, or burnt as incense on charcoal, has been used in ceremony to dispel negativity.

True to False? Test your knowledge of Nettles with this fun quiz at: https://www.athomewithjaniceschofieldeaton.com/stinging-nettles/quiz-test-your-nettle-knowledge

Nettles for Fiber

Nettles have a long history of use for making fabric and cordage. The following photo, from the National Museum of Denmark, shows nettle cloth remnants from the Bronze Age.

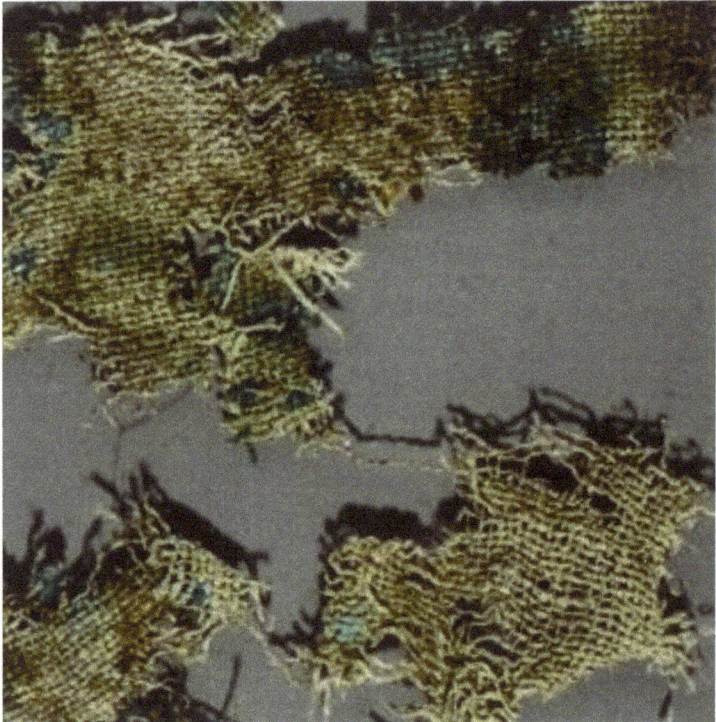

Wartime shortages stimulated the use of nettle for making uniforms and other clothing. According to Dr. Christopher's *Herbal Legacy*, "During World War I, the German Empire, plagued by textile shortages, used nettles as a substitute for cotton. Uniforms from captured German soldiers were found to be 85% nettle fiber."

The durable and adaptable nettle is being resurrected today as a fashion item. Nettles harvested from Prince Charles Highgrove Estate were woven into fabric and utilized in high fashion designs by London sustainable design duo Vin and Omi.[42] (To see photos of their designs, visit: https://fashionunited. uk/news/fashion/nettles-with-royal-roots-hit-the-london-cat-walks/2019091845314).

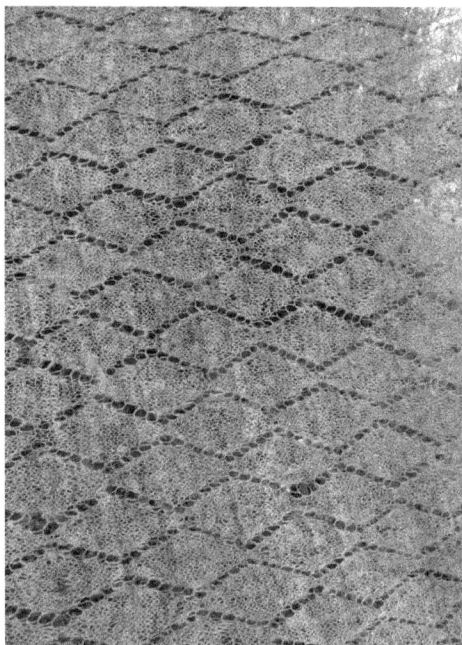

You might expect nettle fibers to be rough in texture and unattractive. But a visitor, Don Graves, displayed a handmade shawl he had bought in Nepal that was exquisite and soft.

According to February 2002 IENICA (Interactive European Network for Industrial Crops and their Applications) newsletter, a European project was starting in 1999 with nettles "...to observe the possibilities for this plant to be cultivated as a raw material for the production of fibres and cellulose using modern methods of plant production and fibre processing." Project partners included textile companies from Germany, Austria, and Italy. IENICA planted two hectares (five acres) of nettles (over 50,000 plants). "After harvest, the dry stems were decorticated by a flax company in Austria and the fibres sent to Germany." IENICA reports that its partners are still busy spinning experimental yarns.

Leimomi Oakes, a textile and fashion historian who writes a blog, the Dreamstress, displays photos of a fairy tale nettle smock that she sewed. Though I've yet to weave nettle clothing, I have created many a ball of nettle (and nettle-fireweed) string for Alaskan bush cabin applications. My favorite method was to collect the nettles in spring after snowmelt. In Alaska, the nettle stalks are compacted by winter snow. In my present New Zealand location, the overwintered stalks remain erect, as shown in the photo (right).

Sara Doyle of Palmer Alaska, in personal communication, wrote: "We've used nettle cordage for a number of items and have been impressed by how well it holds, even when it is fairly thin. We did cold-smoked salmon over three weeks, and the nettle cordage was so lovely after the smoke-colored it a bit. It also seemed more heat tolerant than basic kitchen cotton twine."

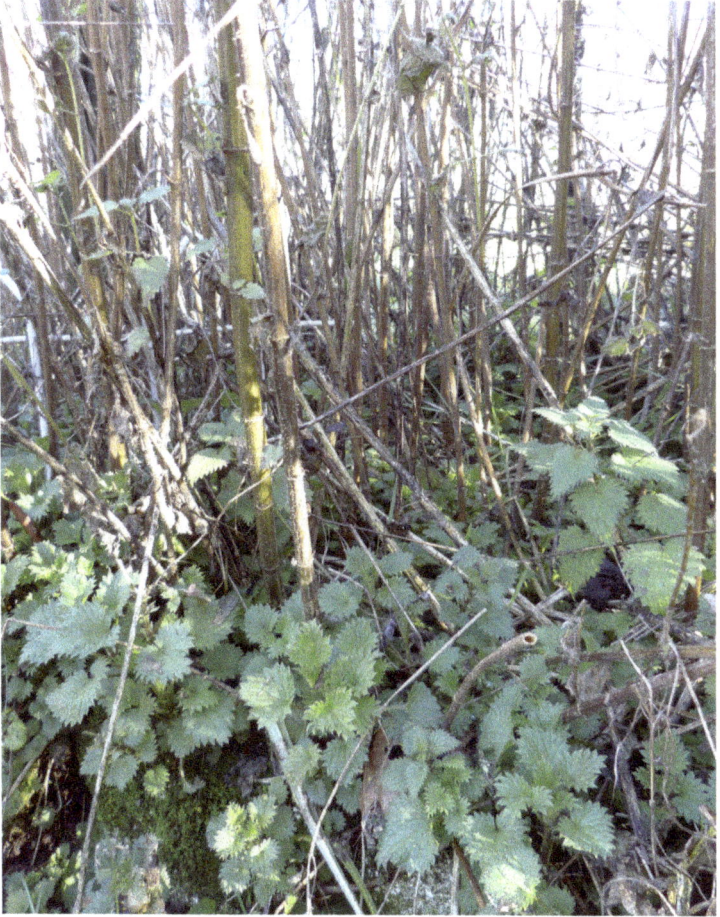

There are various YouTube clips available on making reverse-wrapped nettle cordage.

Readers Notes

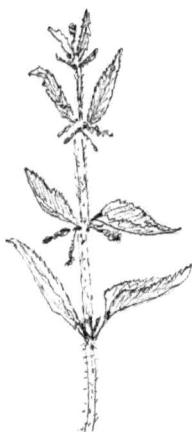

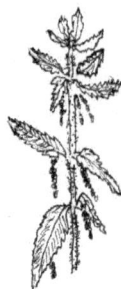

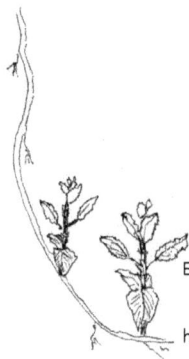

E-mail your new recipes and nettle experiences to:
athomewithjanice@gmail.com
for potential inclusion in the blog:
https://www.athomewithjaniceschofieldeaton.com

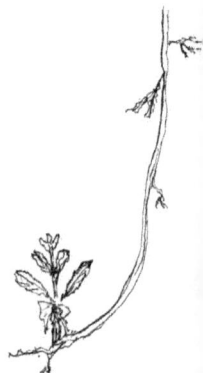

Endnotes

1. Botanical illustration by Prof. Dr. Otto Wilhelm Thomé Flora von Deutschland, Österreich und der Schweiz 1885, Gera, Germany

2. Photographs by Frank Vincentz; © 2000, 2001, 2002 Free Software Foundation, Inc. 51 Franklin St, Fifth Floor, Boston, MA 02110-1301

3. de Lange, P.J. (2020): Urtica ferox Fact Sheet). New Zealand Plant Conservation Network. https://www. nzpcn.org.nz/flora/species/*urtica-ferox*/ (accessed online 30/12/20).

4. Mrs. M. Grieve, *A Modern Herbal* (New York: Dover Publications, Inc., 1931, reprint, 1971, p. 574

5. Staff of the L. H. Bailey Hortorium, *Hortus Third* (N. Y.: Macmillan Publishing Company, 1976), pp. 168-169, 872.

6. Bob Flaws, *The Book of Jook: Chinese Medicinal Porridges—A Healthy Alternative to the Typical Western Breakfast* (Boulder, Co., Blue Poppy Press, 1995, p. 8)

7. Michael Moore, *Medicinal Plants of the Pacific West* (Santa Fe, N. M., Red Crane Books, 1993), p. 189-190

8. Grieve, Mrs. M. *A Modern Herbal*. New York, New York: Dover Publications, Inc., 1971.

9. Dawson, Adele. *Health, Happiness and the Pursuit of Herbs*. Brattleboro, Vermont: The Steven Greene Press, 1980.

10. Stern, Gai. *Australian Weeds*. Sydney, New South Wales: Harper and Rowe, 1986.

11. Treben, Maria. *Health Through God's Pharmacy*. Steyr: Wilhelm Ennsthaler, 1983.

12. Michael Moore, *Medicinal Plants of the Pacific West* (Santa Fe, N. M., Red Crane Books, 1993), p. 188

13. H. N. Obretenova, D. Keysova, K. Petrova, "*Akad. Nauk*," Izv. Inst. Khranere, 1973, 11:5

14. "Silicon Protects Against Aluminum," *MediHerb Monitor*, June 1944, 9:2.

15. N.Bisset, *Herbal Drugs and Phytopharmaceuticals* (Stuttgart, Germany: CRC Press, 1994), pp. 502-7.

16. Susanne Fischer-Rizzi, *Medicine of the Earth* (Portland, Oregon: Rudra Press, 1996), p 257

17. Michael Moore, *Medicinal Plants of the Pacific West* (Santa Fe, N. M., Red Crane Books, 1993), p. 188

18. P. Musette, A. Galelli, et. al., "Urtica dioica Agglutinin, a V-Beta 8.3-Specific Superantigen, Prevents the Development of the Systemic Lupus Erythematosus-like Pathology of MRL, 1pr/1pr Mice," Eur. J. Immunol., August 1996, 26:1707-11.

19. Carole Fischer and Gilian Painter, *Materia Medica of Western Herbs for The Southern Hemisphere* (Auckland, New Zealand: Gilian Painter, 1996), p. 237

20. Michael Moore, *Medicinal Plants of the Mountain West* (Santa Fe, N. M.: Red Crane Books, 1993), p. 114.

21. T. Krezeski, et al. "Combined Extracts of *Urtica dioica* and *Pygeum africanum* in the Treatment of Benign Prostatic Hyperplasia: Double-blind Comparison of Two Doses," Clin. Ther. 15 (6): 1011-20.

22. Carole Fischer and Gilian Painter, *Materia Medica of Western Herbs for The Southern Hemisphere* (Auckland, New Zealand: Gilian Painter, 1996), p. 237.

23. G. Champault, J. C. Patel, A. M. Bonnard, "A Double-blind Trial of an Extract of the Plant *Serenoa repens* in Benign Prostratic Hyperplasia, Br. Journal Clin. Pharmacal 1984: 18: 461-462.

24. James Green, *The Male Herbal* (Freedom, Ca.: The Crossing Press, 1991), p. 104.

25. M. S. Fahim, et. al. "Zinc Treatment for Reduction of Hyperplasia of Prostate." Fed. Proc., 35: 361

26. Dorothy Shepherd, M. D., *A Physician's Posy* (Essex, England: Health Science Press, 1981 (from revised edition of 1969), pp. 210-219.

27. Michael Tierra, C. A., N. D., *Planetary Herbology* (Santa Fe, N. M.: Lotus Press, 1988), p. 35.

28. Juliette de Bairacli Levy, *The Complete Herbal Handbook for Farm and Stable* (London-Boston: Faber and Faber, 1984), pp. 104-105.

29. Research Gate: "Effect of Dietary Nettle Extract on Pig Meat Quality" E. Hanczakowska, Medcyna Weternaryjna 63:(5):525-527, May 2007

30. J. Kolousek, et. al. *"Akad. Zemedel Ved."* Sbornik Ceskoslov, 1954: 27A: 113.

31. Levy, Juliette de Bairacli. *The Complete Herbal Handbook for Farm and Stable.* London-Boston: Faber and Faber, 1984.

32. http://www.henriettesherbal.com/blog/nettle-seed. html

33. Stern, Gai. *Australian Weeds.* Sydney, New South Wales: Harper and Rowe, 1986.

34. Berg, Ed. "Be Nice to Nettles. " Refuge Notebook; Vol. 6, No. 19, 2004, May 14.

35. http://www.monarch.org.nz/monarch/other-species/ factsheets/plants/beginners-guide-to-nettles/, August 14, 2012 (Trust n.d.)

36. Dickey, Delwyn (10 March 2016). "Stinging native plant behind butterfly comeback". *Stuff.* Retrieved 27 Dec 2020

37. https://www.forestandbird.org.nz/resources/ attracting-butterflies-to-garden

38. https://teara.govt.nz, "Monarch Butterflies," Retrieved 19 Jan. 2021

39. https://www.nettles.org.uk, Be Nice to Nettles Week, retrieved 19 Jan, 2021

40. *Urtica* spp.: Ordinary Plants with Extraordinary Properties, Kriegal, Pawlikowska, and Antolak, Molecules. 2018 Jul; 23(7): 1664. Retrieved online 19 Jan 2021

41. http://www.traditionalmusic.co.uk/folk-song-lyrics/
    Cowe_the_Nettle.htm

42. https://www.dezeen.com/2019/09/25/
    vin-omi-prince-charles-nettles-london-fashion-week/

INDEX